"Because I was there when several of these stories were being impressed on Stan's heart, I know that he has not exaggerated or played to emotions.

"It is incredible how alike are we peoples of the world and how much we who have seldom known deprivation have to learn from those who live their lifetimes with it. Charity is the starting point for learning, but I do not think that God will be satisfied, or that we can be, unless we also achieve justice.

"Stan Mooneyham has been entrusted by God with seeing more of the world's hurts than most, not simply for his own understanding but so that he can let the rest of us feel that hurt, too.

"Our spiritual life, and even the part of it that represents our Christ-motivated benevolence, tends to become antiseptic and impersonal. This book helps to make it the hands-on and hearts-on experience it was supposed to be."

-Kenneth L. Wilson

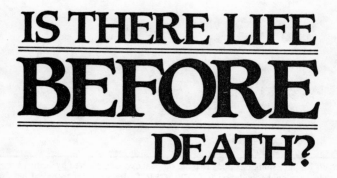

IS THERE LIFE
BEFORE
DEATH?

My Personal Encounters with
the World's Hungry People

STAN MOONEYHAM

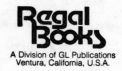

A Division of GL Publications
Ventura, California, U.S.A.

131482

© 1985

Rights for publishing this book in other languages are contracted by Gospel Literature International foundation (GLINT). GLINT also provides technical help for
the adaptation, translation, and publishing of Bible study resources and books in
over 100 languages worldwide. For further information, contact GLINT, Post
Office Box 6688, Ventura, California 93006, U.S.A., or the publisher.

Scripture quotations in this publication are from the following:
KJV—The Authorized King James version
NEB—*The New English Bible.* © The Delegates of the Oxford University Press
1961, 1970. Reprinted by permission.
TLB—*The Living Bible,* Copyright © 1971 by Tyndale House Publishers,
Wheaton, Illinois. Used by permission.

Published by Regal Books
A Division of GL Publications
Ventura, California 93006
Printed in U.S.A.

Library of Congress Cataloging in Publication Data

Mooneyham, W. Stanley (Walter Stanley), 1926-
    Is there life before death?

    1. Developing countries—Economic conditions. 2. Food supply—
Developing countries. 3. Mooneyham, W. Stanley (Walter Stanley), 1926-
4. Missionaries—Developing countries. 5. Missionaries—United States. I.
Title.
HC59.7.M5765 1985   363.8'2'091724   84-29839
ISBN 0-8307-1025-6

To
my spiritual family
at the
Palm Desert
Community Presbyterian Church
and our shepherd,
Dr. Dean W. Miller,
who tenderly provide a
way station
for the healing of
bruised prophets.

Contents

Introduction

Perhaps what follows will mean more to you if I first tell you something of my emotional struggles during 15 years of ministry among the world's dispossessed and disfranchised people.

You need to know that it's a ministry, not a job. It's a spiritual call, not a calculated choice. If it were a self-chosen vocation, I likely would have abandoned it long ago. While it is certainly fulfilling, it is not fun.

During the first few years, I was afraid that I might burn out emotionally. I didn't know—and still don't—how much exposure to the hurts of others a human being can handle. I talked with a couple of doctors to see how they managed rubbing shoulders on a daily basis with suffering and death. They didn't have a formula either.

I understood enough psychology to know that sustained overstimulation of the nervous system is destructive. Human emotions are fragile, and I was pretty sure that feelings not dealt with can lie inside you like a ticking bomb waiting to explode. All in all, I didn't feel too comfortable about it.

But as much as I wanted to avoid emotional overload, I was more afraid of compassion fatigue. The Bible calls it growing "weary in well doing" (Gal. 6:9). Simply stated, I wanted to be spared the curse of cold professionalism. I'm not talking about competence here. I'm talking about an attitude that allows us to change people into statistics and a ministry into a job.

I'm talking about what some derelict must have felt when on the wall of a rescue mission he wrote this bit of graffiti:

> Organized charity
>   carefully iced;
> In the name of a careful,
>   statistical Christ.

What I was looking for was the balance between emotional composure and disabling compassion. Somewhere, I reasoned, there must be a livable middle ground between being hardhearted and soft-headed. I've never had trouble weeping with those who weep. My emotional identification with the dying country of Cambodia where I had spent so much time was so total that when it fell to the Communists in 1975, I went into a grief-induced depression so deep that I had to be medically treated for an extended period.

That experience scared me. So much so, in fact, that I seriously started looking for answers that would help me function without becoming a basket case on the one hand or a Christian bureaucrat on the other.

I didn't have to look far. For me, the answers are found in the life and ministry of Jesus, but they are not a magic formula. I am having to learn them one day at a time.

First, I accept that it's OK to go ahead and feel my feelings, whatever the risk. That cuts across the grain of American culture. We are masters at masking our feelings, having been taught the art from childhood. I heard it again the other day: "I know I shouldn't feel this way, but . . . . "

What self-deception we engage in! We feel human emotions and deny the feelings. When Jesus was throwing the commercial interests out of the Temple, I don't hear Him saying, "I know I shouldn't feel angry, but—" Or when castigating the Pharisees, He doesn't piously say, "I know I shouldn't despise these rascals, but—" At the tomb of Lazarus He openly wept over the loss of His friend. And from the cross, He felt and practiced forgiveness.

I find no evidence that Jesus indulged His feelings, but He certainly did not mask them. He simply felt them as an honest response to each situation.

That's my model. Yet I find that it's painful to volunteer for emotional wounding over and over again. There are times when I want to draw back from feeling. I am not a masochist who gets pleasure from pain, but neither do I want to become a bundle of scar tissue with no nerve endings.

Speaking of his decision not to allow Vietnamese boat refugees to land in his country, the Prime Minister of Singapore, Lee Kuan Yew, said, "You have to develop callouses on your heart; otherwise, you will bleed to death."

His statement chills me. I think we do not bleed enough. It is too easy for me to slip into apathy to worry about bleeding to death. I worry that I will not bleed at all. And I know that quiet acquiescence will never call forth the sacrifice necessary to change the status quo.

So I cry and I rage. Injustice gets me white-hot angry. A starving child moves me to tears. Sometimes I bleed.

And what about the scar tissue with dead nerve endings? Mother Teresa helped me with that one day as we were talking in Calcutta. I shared with her the discomfort of feeling like a yo-yo—out and back, out and back. Helping hungry and homeless people one day; back in my comfortable, affluent world the next. Only partially in jest, I said, "I think I would be more comfortable if I took the vow of poverty and came out here to join you."

Wisely and gently, she replied, "You must allow God to make you a bridge without asking you."

As I thought about that, I decided that since God has called me to be a bridge between two worlds, I would simply have to depend upon Him to heal the emotional wounds inflicted in the world of hunger so that I might function without guilt in my other world. Surprisingly, I am learning that His healing is without scar tissue. He heals us that we may be wounded again. So until and unless I see it differently, I will go ahead and feel my feelings.

The other thing I am learning is to accept my human limitations. Being able to do so little in the face of such staggering need invariably leaves me frustrated. Interviewers add to my feelings of helplessness with the constant query: "Do you think you are making a dent in the hunger problem?"

The only honest answer is no, but I have to say something else. It usually goes like this: "That beggars the real question, which is, 'Am I doing what I can do as one person?' If my answer to that is yes, then I am able to sleep at night."

Too many are afflicted with statistical paralysis. They are immobilized by the overwhelming and staggering numbers—what we call the "hunger problem," the "refugee problem" or the "poverty problem."

I don't work on problems; I help people. Again, Jesus is my model. He did not heal every sick person in Palestine nor did He feed all the hungry. He did not set right every injustice, nor did He spend His every waking moment attempting to do those things. He slept and went on retreats. He attended parties and led seminars. He lived life in its ordinary dimensions and I believe He expects me to do the same.

But—and here is the test of my faithfulness—He

never turned away from helping anyone who came within the scope of His awareness. I can do that. So can you.

For me, that knowledge brings international problems down to manageable proportions. I no longer have as a personal goal the feeding of a hungry world or the elimination of poverty as a system. I don't know why God Himself hasn't done away with hunger and poverty, but since He hasn't, I will not get statistical paralysis over my inability to do the whole job.

I will make my personal contribution in both areas, doing what I am able to do in any given circumstance, and then I will sleep without guilt. I don't know of any other way to maintain emotional balance.

Years ago, I came across a bit of doggerel written by the British missionary pioneer, C.T. Studd. Nurtured in the lap of comfort, educated at Eton and Cambridge and a sports hero to the cricket-loving British public, young Studd created quite a stir in the secular world of his day by renouncing wealth and position to follow Christ to the regions beyond. When he died on the mission field in 1931, he had spent 46 years in three separate missionary careers in China, India and Africa.

The motivation of his life, which I have sought to make my own, is found in these four lines:

Some wish to live within the sound
　　Of church or chapel bell,
I want to run a rescue shop
　　Within a yard of hell.

If, as you read these stories, you sometimes feel you are standing on the brink yourself, the people in the stories would identify with your feelings. That's where they live out their daily existence. From that razor edge of survival, they cannot afford the luxury of an academic debate over whether or not there is life *after* death. That argument is reserved for the well-fed, adequately-housed, fully-clothed, comfortably-fixed Christian who has the time and energy for theological gymnastics.

The question asked by those you'll read about on these pages is more basic. They would like to know, "Will we have a chance to live before we have to die?"

For me, and perhaps for them, there is some comfort in the knowledge that God hears the question and seeks to send an affirmative answer through those who are willing to give, to go and to serve.

Here am I, Lord, send me.

1

The Cross at the Edge of Hell

Egypt

The smoldering fires on the mountains of garbage lit the darkness as they leaped into tongues of flame, giving a rosy hue to the smoky pall hanging over the surrealistic setting. Shadowy figures moved in and out of the light as scavenging dogs snarled their way around the slopes.

The scene reminded me of a Salvador Dali painting.

Except for the smell. The smell of Cairo's burning leftovers was not an illusion. It was real.

Acrid. Pungent. Penetrating. Just the way, I thought, it must have smelled in the Valley of Hinnom outside Jerusalem where, in ancient times, a fire was kept burning constantly to consume the waste of animals slaughtered for temple sacrifices.

It was from this place of perpetual fire that Jewish writers acquired their word *Gehenna,* which first was used to mean "the entrance to hell" and later hell itself.

Yes, I said, that's what it's like.

Gehenna.

And the family of Sa'ad Abed el Said Suher, with whom I had spent the last three days, lived at the bottom of those burning mounds. They lived, I mused, within a yard of hell.

Actually, the name of the place is Zarayeb and it is home to over 10,000 people, all of whom make their living recycling what Cairo's 10 million inhabitants throw away. They represent about one-third of the city's garbage collectors. The rest live in three other settlements, the largest of which has a population of 14,000.

During my time at Zarayeb, I learned a great deal about how a subculture lives. I discovered that what I thought was merely a "garbage dump" was actually a town with a life, character, structure and system all its own.

I gained a deep appreciation of the people, of their ability to organize themselves, of their struggles to beat the odds, and especially of their hopes and dreams for themselves and their children.

Among them, I met people I was proud to own as brothers and sisters. Like Sa'ad and his family.

From the moment I stepped into their little compound, I felt a kinship with this sensitive man who has worked in the garbage dump since he was 10 years old. At least that's how old he thinks he was when a compassionate uncle brought him to Cairo.

His father had been a mechanic in Tahta, a poverty-stricken village in the upper Nile Valley about 600 miles from Egypt's capital city. But, faced with little food for his family and no future for his son, he agreed when his wife's brother, who had a garbage route in Cairo, offered to take young Sa'ad into "the business" with him.

The business, I learned, is a hard, tough one from which every person involved hopes ultimately to escape.

As Sa'ad and I sat down to talk, bottles of warm Pepsi-Cola appeared from somewhere and were placed in the visitors' hands. Since there is no electricity or ice in

Zarayeb, the fact that the drinks were warm didn't bother me as much as seeing them uncapped, not knowing when, where or by whom it had been done. But to have refused this generous act of hospitality would have been unthinkable; so I wiped the top with my own dirty hand and apprehensively sipped the contents.

A brief visual survey of the compound confirmed that life for a collector of garbage is very basic indeed. The area was about 30 feet square and served as home for two families—Sa'ad's and that of his sister who had come from Tahta to Cairo and married after Sa'ad established his own collection route.

At the back of the compound was a pig pen with a population of 27.

Scrap sheets of metal separated Sa'ad's compound from those of his neighbors. Everything was open to the sky except for two small covered huts in opposite corners where the families slept. The rest of the living was done in the open. The huts were built of scrap—bits of tin, cardboard, cloth, wood. Virtually everything in the compound, from cooking utensils to clothing, seemed to be what someone else had thrown away. Including, I was sure, the bench where we sat and drank warm Pepsi as we talked.

"What are some of your problems?" I asked this self-taught and barely literate man whose age we had established at somewhere between 30 and 35.

His answer is a revelation in itself: "This whole life is a problem. What do you want to know about?" indicating that I needed to be more specific.

"Well, the police," I said. "What kinds of problems do you have with the police?"

"Sometimes they are very kind and leave me alone," he said softly. "But sometimes they arrest me because I have no identity card. They keep me for a day or two until they make some kind of report. Then I lose work. I can't get a card because I haven't done my military service, but I can't go into the army because I can't leave my wife and children here."

It is a dilemma for which he has no answer except a shrug of the shoulders. I am beginning to understand his statement, "This whole life is a problem."

"What about your health?" I ask. The handling of garbage, the long hours and backbreaking labor, the living conditions all seem designed to contribute to sickness. "Is your health bad?"

Another insight, this time from Pastor Boushra Assaad, my interpreter, whose Coptic Evangelical Presbyterian Church is starting a social work here.

"He doesn't know how to answer your question since he wouldn't recognize anything apart from a serious sickness," he explains. "He just thanks God that he is strong enough to work.

"But I can tell you that sickness among the children is a major problem," Pastor Boushra continues. "There are no health services here and the nearest hospital is five miles away. The children have skin diseases, worms, eye infections and pneumonia. The water is polluted and rats carry disease from hut to hut. I estimate that 10 to 15 children die here every day."

He repeats to Sa'ad what he has told me, and the man nods his head. "Two of our children died," he said simply. I see three others playing around the compound. The oldest looks about eight and the youngest is just walking.

Most of the children in Zarayeb work the donkey carts with their fathers, walking up long flights of stairs and carrying garbage down. Sa'ad works alone. He insists that his son go to school, even though it's a four-mile round-trip walk every day.

"I will never allow my children to work in the garbage!" he tells me emphatically.

Pastor Boushra points out that the things I am asking about are only symptoms of a deeper and larger problem—the garbage collection system itself. Most of the people will always struggle just to survive because they cannot change their status within the system. For the most part, they are illiterate peasants who come from upper Egypt hoping to find jobs in Cairo. But lacking skills, they simply drift to the bottom of the jobless pool and end up as human cogs in the garbage-collecting system.

The system itself is privately organized, unregulated except by unwritten rules among those who control it. These "bosses," usually from families who managed to graduate from the carts, stake out territories in the city, each of which has several hundred apartments and houses. The boss charges each household 30 cents a week, but most often the collector sees none of this. The money simply guarantees that the boss will keep the system working smoothly and prevent other cart operators from competing.

If it seems like protection money, it must be admitted that both the householders and collectors are afraid of the bosses and no one cares to challenge their right to collect the fee. Nonetheless, it must be said also that the system works, and that makes it worthwhile for all concerned, including the government which has been relieved of one more administrative function.

If the boss is humane, he may give the collector five cents a month for each client, but most are not so kind. In fact, if an apartment dweller gives the collector or his children anything of value, the boss is supposed to be told about it so he can decide if the collector may keep it or turn it over to him.

But the outside boss is not the only one with whom Sa'ad must deal. There is a boss who owns the land on which all the garbage collectors are squatters. He must be satisfied, too. The rent on Sa'ad's compound is $200 a year. By virtue of owning the land, the boss gets one-third of the pigs that grow fat on the garbage Sa'ad feeds them. He is also the middleman for selling the rest of the porkers, taking a substantial cut of the profits, since Sa'ad with his minimal literacy doesn't know how to handle that kind of business.

Then there are the bosses who, through other middlemen, buy what Sa'ad salvages from his daily collections. As I began to understand the system, it seemed to me that, as in so many other parts of the world, it was calculated to victimize and exploit those who put the most labor into it.

At the end of a day which begins at 5:30 A.M., Sa'ad may have cleared between 50 cents and a dollar. The higher amount would be possible only if the garbage contained any "treasure"—a pair of shoes, a toy or broken household items that could be repaired. He told me that once he found a gold watch valued at nearly $2,000. Being an honest man, he returned it and was given a $25 reward.

But that happened only once. On each of the days I was there, he averaged less than 50 cents. I watched as the weary donkeys turned into the open gates of the compound at 2:00 in the afternoon, having pulled the primitive little cart over a 14-mile course. Two obviously streetwise cats jumped nimbly to the top of the loaded cart and started fighting over a choice morsel.

The children greeted their father with squeals and hugs, the way children all over the world greet fathers coming home from work.

Sa'ad unhitched the donkeys and they immediately proceeded to wallow in a dustbath, relieved that another day was over. But for the man, there was still much to do. He tipped the cart, allowing the garbage to spill out the back into the compound. The flies descended like one of

Moses' plagues, claiming the garbage as their own.

Oblivious to the swarm around them, the man and his wife started the sorting process. Their hands flew as they handled each scrap, separating according to final disposition. Food scraps went into a bucket for feeding the pigs. A pile was started for tin cans. Another for bottles. One for plastic containers. One for paper scraps. And a final one for the residue which could not be sold or used. It was the smallest of all.

During the sorting process, a woman comes by who regularly buys the plastic containers. There is a bit of good-humored haggling as she says, "You keep all the best stuff for yourself and sell me only the junk. It's the same the world over."

Finally, the pile is weighed on primitive scales and a deal is struck. Sa'ad turns back to help his wife who has never allowed her hands to stop the sorting. There are no treasures today at the end of the hour-and-a-half process.

Although he is tired, we sit down on the bench to talk again. I want to try to get inside the man, to understand something of what he thinks and feels. Gently, I ask what it is like to be at the bottom of the ladder and be looked down on by other people.

He hesitates a moment. I have touched a nerve.

"The first year I worked with my uncle, I was very ashamed," Sa'ad admits. "I didn't want to go to the people. I would come back every day feeling depressed. But, finally, I got used to it and it doesn't bother me any more. I accept this as my trade, my way to live, and I am not ashamed of it.

"In fact, since I became a Christian I am able to thank God for this work because that is why I am still living."

As I look at his face, I see a man at peace. Peace—just at the edge of hell.

But I know this is not the experience of most of the

people who live in Zarayeb. Pastor Boushra confirms that psychological problems abound. Different people handle them in different ways, he tells me. The pressure is so great on some they become mentally ill. Some turn to criminal activity, using the anonymity found in Zarayeb to cover their crimes. Still others numb themselves with drugs and alcohol.

"Almost everyone in this place uses drugs," Sa'ad agrees. "It is the only way to forget who they are and what they do. I myself used drugs until I became a Christian. Now those things like smoking, drinking and drugs are . . . rubbish!"

I smile at his use of the word for it seems incongruous in this situation. But I fully understand what he means.

Sa'ad tells me he became a Christian on July 23, 1975. He remembers the date well. A layman from Pastor Boushra's church, Boulas Goda, a converted drug dealer, came and preached the gospel to those who formerly bought his drugs. Sa'ad was one of the early converts.

As the former drug dealer began to make regular trips to the garbage dump to share his new faith, more people turned to Christ and he saw the need for starting a church. Pastor Boushra agreed to go and preach one Sunday. He told me what he found: "After the service, I went to visit a very sick 15-year-old girl. She was lying on the ground, barely able to move. I told them I'd come back the next day and take her to the hospital, but when I went back she was dead. I was very upset. The people told me that children were always dying here.

"They are malnourished and get sick so easily. Mostly they eat what we call 'white cheese' which is milk sealed in a can and allowed to sit for a long time until the curdled milk has separated from the whey. They dip their bread in this and sometimes they have a few vegetables. Only on very special occasions do they get meat.

"I went back and told my elders about the suffering people and they agreed our church should do something. But what to do? Yes, I'd like to deliver Jesus to them, but what kind of Jesus could they understand?

"It is not enough for me to bring words only," Pastor Boushra says emotionally. "God never intended for us to sit idle while the restless poor struggle to survive. I have to get involved with their hunger, their diseases, their illiteracy. So we decided to help all the people, Christians and Muslims alike."

Less than 10 percent of the people are Muslims because the Muslim religion does not allow them to work with swine.

Pastor Boushra believes that the gospel is the best hope for changing the lives of the garbage workers, and he has some pretty convincing evidence to back up his belief.

"When the people accept Christ and stop gambling, drinking and taking drugs," he says, "they are able to save some money. They put their children in school and make a down payment on a small piece of land outside the garbage dump. They start to build a simple house one brick at a time. While all this may take four or five years, for the first time they begin to live with hope."

At least 25 Christian families have moved away through this method.

On the way to church on Sunday, we stop at the home of one of them. Boulas Shinouda worked in the garbage for over 20 years. He and his younger brother, Gabriel, built this place themselves and started a business selling reinforcing iron. The house has four rooms and is clean. There are no flies even though it is less than a mile from the garbage dump. All four children go to school.

The only other way out of the garbage dump is to become a boss, using threats and intimidation. I agree with Pastor Boushra that the gospel is better.

The church in Zarayeb looks like everything else there. It is a hut made from scrap. Scrap benches with one or two rusty folding chairs sit on the dirt floor. Two recycled lanterns hang from the low ceiling.

A cross over the doorway is pieced together from scrap plastic. It isn't very artistic, but then I remember that neither was the one raised on Jerusalem's garbage dump, Golgotha.

Packed into the 10-by-25-foot church are about 90 people, men on one side and women on the other. Some sit on the ground for lack of a bench. As we arrive, they are singing in Arabic a rhythmic song accompanied by hand-clapping and the tinkling sound of finger cymbals. Some of the men weep as they sing: "The voice comes from heaven . . . the voice of love . . . I'll never forget you . . . I'll never leave you, my son . . . the sun will be shining after the clouds."

The sermon is punctuated with spontaneous responses from the men, who make up more than half the congregation. The service ends with mass prayer as all the people pray individual prayers at the same time. Then they sing a hymn, "I'm not worthy, Lord, of all the good things you have done for me," followed by the Lord's Prayer.

As I step out into the sunlight, I look up at the smoking mounds of garbage and back again at the humble little chapel with the recycled cross over the door. The people coming out still have the joy of the Lord in their faces and their voices.

Somehow it doesn't seem right. Why should they be happy? But then a happy thought strikes me. Why not? Heaven begins, after all, just at the edge of hell.

2

Catapulting into the Twentieth Century

Kenya

Now that I think back, the lift-off from Kitale early that morning should have tipped me off about the kind of day it was going to be.

As we drove onto the grass strip in Kenya's "white highlands," we could barely make out the helicopter through the swirling fog. It was not, at least from ground level, one of your better mornings for flying. After a brief discussion of the options—and because the time schedule for the day was pressing—we decided at least to test the thickness of the fog layer.

When we were belted in, our pilot, Van Smith, started flipping switches. In a few minutes, the motor atop the Bell Jet Ranger roared alive.

Van's intention was to climb maybe a hundred feet to see if we could spot the sun which should be rising about now. If not, we'd descend and wait. But at less than a hundred feet the ground disappeared in the fog and there was still no open sky above.

Since the small grass strip from which we had taken off was surrounded by trees and now lost in the fog, the safest way to go was up. The decision made, we went up.

Up into the soup.

I'm not sure how long I held my breath (at least, I don't recall breathing), but it wasn't until the altimeter showed 500 feet that we broke into the clear. I punctuated the event with an audible, tension-breaking "whew!"

Van, who formerly flew for the Marines, grinned and turned the craft northwest toward the Ugandan border into one of those never-to-be-forgotten days.

We left the foggy area and, from clearer air, soon watched the terrain change from lush green fields to reddish sand that produced little more than scrub and thornbushes. Flowing streams dwindled into dry riverbeds, and neat cement block houses gave way to little native *bomas*.

The 40-minute flight was a journey centuries back in time. The people we were going to visit—the Pokot—are still in the early Iron Age. They still do not use the wheel. Their name means "hospitable," but the British called them *Suk*.

When the colonizers first penetrated their remote area, they asked the people, "What is your name?" Trying to appear unworthy of the attention of the foreigners so they would go away, the people replied, "Oh, we're *suk* (dead logs)." What they were really saying was "Don't bother us; just leave us alone." But the British thought that *suk* was the name of the tribe and it stuck until recent years.

As we flew over the rutted, dusty road we spotted the four Land Rovers beneath us carrying the rest of our team. We figured they would arrive at Kiwawa about two hours after us. They had left well before daylight in order to make the rendezvous.

After dropping us in a cloud of dust at the Kiwawa feeding center, Van took off immediately for the return trip to pick up the rest of our team, including actress/singer

Carol Lawrence with whom I was taping a television documentary. That's the way the day started, and the sun was still less than an hour above the horizon.

We had just sat down under a tent for a bite of breakfast when an army patrol came barreling down the dirt road yelling that a thousand Karamajong cattle raiders from Uganda were attacking the village of Losom, six miles away, and shooting up the place. It was an extremely treacherous situation. Our convoy would be coming down that road in less than an hour. Among others in the vehicles were missionaries Mike and Linda Courtney and their two children.

The convoy might be headed straight into an ambush!

Missionary Dick Hamilton and I were not quite sure what we could do, but it took only a few minutes for us to decide what we could *not* do, and that was stay at Kiwawa and allow events to simply play themselves out. If we could burst our way through the fighting at Losom, we would almost certainly be able to intercept the convoy and prevent a possible massacre.

The other possibility also had to be considered. We might get shot.

Just a week before, a Roman Catholic priest was fired on as he drove a vehicle down that road. Two of his passengers were killed. The border between Uganda and Kenya in the Karapokot area was not one of the world's safe places.

The decision was virtually a self-made one dictated by the circumstances. Dick and I turned to each other and said almost simultaneously, "Let's go!"

My son, Eric, a documentary photographer with whom I had shared other anxious moments like this one, was the first one in the Toyota Land Cruiser. He was followed by Diane Messik, a nurse from Canton, Ohio, who brought along her medical kit, knowing there would be casualties. If there were, Diane would know what to do.

Justin Sylvestre, a young volunteer with the mission, and our television crewmen, Dick Davies and Steve Berry, climbed in, and we headed out. Dick Hamilton drove while I stayed on the radio trying to raise Van in the helicopter.

Some 30 or 40 Pokot warriors were strung out along the narrow road toward Losom. Dressed only in their *shukas*—a cloth or animal skin tied over one shoulder—and carrying spears and bows and arrows, they looked fragile and helpless against the automatic weapons carried by the cattle raiders. Nonetheless, they told us they were going to try to recover the cattle. Brave and noble as the act was, it turned out to be futile for most and fatal for some.

Even before arriving at Losom, we could hear the sharp crack of gunfire about 200 to 300 yards off the road. The raiding party was pulling back into the bush as we drove into the village, now deserted except for a dozen or so Kenya soldiers and police. No danger of ambush now.

The Karamajong attackers had left behind two of their dead, one of whom had been the leader, apparently a deserter from the Ugandan army, still wearing his uniform. The raiders took along with them other bodies (bearers accompany each raiding party to remove the dead) and nearly 2,000 head of Pokot cattle. The only animal left was a cow that had broken a leg by falling into a ravine. The raid was a devastating blow to the struggling villagers at Losom.

The Pokot casualties numbered over 50, most of them occurring when young warriors took their primitive weapons in pursuit of the Karamajong who had left an armed rear guard. It was scant comfort to the grieving, impoverished Pokot families to learn that the raiders themselves had been ambushed by the Ugandan militia as they crossed the border returning home, losing about 100 men. The people at Losom had been pushed back to square one.

Cattle rustling among the nomadic tribes of East Africa is not a new practice. Even though the Karamajong, Pokot, Turkana, Toposa, Bume, Dinka and other nomadic peoples are tribal cousins, stealing cattle has been a deadly game among them for centuries.

A man's wealth and status in the community are determined by the number of cattle he owns. In good times, a wealthy man might have up to 5,000 head of cattle. Cows and goats provide life's basic necessities—skins for wearing, horns for carrying rancid butter on long treks, milk and blood for drinking and meat for eating at feasts and ceremonial occasions.

Rebecca Cherona, a development worker and a Pokot herself, told me about the people's love affair with cattle. "The main topic of conversations when the men meet in the evenings is their cows," she said. "They tell and retell stories of encounters with wild animals. They make up songs about their cattle possessing special qualities. A white bull, for example, will have his praises sung in the most picturesque language. Or a bull with the biggest horns. Or a cow that gives a lot of milk, or one with beautiful spots.

"The more special cattle a man owns, the more songs he can make up, which in turn increases his esteem in the minds of others. The larger his herd, the more wives a man can acquire because those cattle mean security.

"The whole society revolves around cattle," she recounted. "For generations, life has ebbed and flowed across these plains as the people search for grass and water for their cows and goats.

"Cattle are a way of life," she concluded.

And as in America's old West, where there are cattle, there are also cattle rustlers. But if the practice of raiding is ancient, the methods are strictly twentieth century. That is part of the evil legacy of Uganda's mad former dictator, Idi Amin, to his country and East Africa. When he was overthrown in 1979, elements of his disintegrating army in the anarchic north blew open an armory and 12,000 modern weapons and two million rounds of ammunition spilled out across the countryside into the hands of primitive people. In one day, they went from bows and arrows to automatic AK-47s, machine guns and grenade launchers.

Since most of these weapons remain in the hands of lawless bands that roam across northern Uganda and often penetrate into Kenya, the Pokot people are being constantly victimized. And though the larger, stronger and more numerous Karamajong now victimize the Pokot, one must remember that they themselves have often been the victims. Even in Uganda itself, the sophisticated and progressive people in the south rarely understand their more primitive citizens in the northern provinces.

Not only does a distance of a few hundred miles separate them. So do culture, life-style and time. Centuries, in fact. Stories circulate in the capital city, Kampala, about "those savages in the deserts up north." Some are probably true; many are fabrications.

It is true that the land is semiarid and the vegetation sparse, but Karamoja is far from being a desert. The Karamajong are primitive and they wear little clothing, but they are not savages.

In fact, their society remained relatively stable for centuries until the mid-1970s when Amin decided the people should become "civilized." He wanted it to happen almost overnight. The trauma of being catapulted from the Iron Age into the twentieth century was destabilizing, to say the least.

Traditionally, when the people wear anything at all,

they cover themselves with animal skins. Even though disease is spread by the hordes of flies attracted by the animal fat which must be rubbed on the hides to keep them supple, the skins are highly practical in a place where every other plant is a thornbush.

Without considering that the thorns would tear them to shreds in no time, Idi Amin wanted the people to wear regular clothes. So an order went out to put trousers on the men and skirts on the women. Publicly, there was some compliance. Many villages acquired just two sets of clothes, one for men and one for women. Anytime a visit to a government post was required, the person going would don the appropriate outfit!

Thus the people observed the letter of the law while thumbing their noses at its spirit. To see a woman in a dress was such a rare sight, the people took to calling such persons "Idi Amin."

Out in the bush, nothing changed.

In one particularly grim episode, Amin sent his soldiers throughout the region on "hunting parties" with orders to shoot on sight those who refused to give up their animal skins and loin cloths. Hundreds of Karamajong were massacred.

Additionally, in order to supply meat to Amin's Libyan friends, his soldiers decimated the cattle herds by either stealing or forcing the people to sell their cattle at shamefully low prices. Although one would never credit the Karamajong with being gentle souls, it is little wonder that they have lashed out at whoever is nearby in retaliation for the injustices that have been inflicted on them in recent years.

At Losom, we had been witnesses to one of the latest of these deadly eruptions. It was the climax of a devastating chain of events: (1) The introduction of automatic weapons, which escalated the violence and further destabilized the society; (2) violence and anarchy then forced many people to leave their traditional grazing lands; (3) drought made it necessary for the people to bring their herds to the few places where water and grass were still available, making them even more vulnerable to raids; (4) the theft of cattle and their death from drought, which reduced many families to absolute poverty; and (5) the lack of rain, which prevented the planting of such usual grain crops as sorghum, millet and maize.

All of this had resulted in dislocation, disease and death affecting some two million people.

The Associated Christian Churches of Kenya, through the team at Kiwawa, were feeding a thousand people each day at that one location. At least 20 percent of the children we saw were badly malnourished. Some of the women walk four to five hours to get their children the special diet of *mboga* (greens), *nyama* (meat) and *ugali* (corn mush) with either rice or beans.

One problem facing the missionaries was the increasing number of deserted children. It was a new phenomenon among the Pokot, who are a very family-oriented people. Though the number of parents abandoning their children was still comparatively small (eight mothers and five fathers), that was eight times what it was the previous year.

Rebecca Cherono, the Pokot social worker, explained that mothers or fathers leave their children only when they are overwhelmed by events and are unable to cope. Now the world seems to be coming down on top of their heads.

If desertion seems heartless, it must be viewed through charitable eyes that understand the circumstances. It may be the last desperate act of love by parents who, having suffered every other indignity with their families, cannot watch helplessly as one or more of their children dies. Saving the child is their first concern.

I think I understood it all a little better as I watched a mother, her eyes brimming with apprehension, take the one piece of cloth she had been wearing and tuck it around her two-year-old child. The mother was left with only her beads and a cattle skin apron.

The father stood by, looking concerned and helpless, as fathers often do. The child was lying on a wooden table that wobbled on the uneven dirt floor, breathing spasmodically, tiny feet cold to the touch. A plastic tube from his scalp led to a bottle tied to the thatched roof of the shelter. The missionary nurse had done her best. She would know in a few hours if it had been enough.

When little Potomoi's parents brought him in that morning, he had pneumonia, was badly dehydrated and was showing the symptoms of measles. Inserting the IV was a problem; the child's arms were so wasted that the nurse could not find a vein. She had to shave one side of the baby's head, put a rubber band around the scalp and gently slap the skin to make a vein stand out, and then, after a couple of frustrating unsuccessful attempts, work in the needle there. The reassuring drip-drip of glucose and penicillin finally began.

The father had been a victim of Ugandan raiders two months earlier. His brother and 15 neighbors were killed, and he himself had lost all his cattle. He confided through a translator: "I heard people say that God answers prayer. So last night I prayed."

An outsider standing by gently said to the mother, "I have a four-year-old. I can feel for you and your husband."

Not taking her eyes from her baby, the mother replied, "Everyone who has a child feels the same things."

3

Forgotten Refugees, Abandoned Brothers

Burma

"Three months ago the soldiers came and killed 20 people in my village, eight of them my relatives. Then we walked for a week and came here."

Here was the refugee village of Kyoe Waing at the edge of a rugged jungle on the banks of Asia's second longest river, the Salween.

The young woman telling me her story is from the Karen (accent on the last syllable, Ka-*ren*) tribe. She sits on the split bamboo floor of a little shack that serves the newly settled village as both Buddhist temple and clinic. She awaits treatment along with some 30 other refugees.

Her 18-month-old baby, too listless to whimper, leans against her breast and starts to nurse. The mother's 17 years have been filled already with a lifetime of tragedy. When the soldiers came and destroyed her village she was still in shock from the death of her husband. He had died of cholera.

Her name, Ka The Htoo, means "golden medicine." If medicine were available for her baby or if there had been any for her husband, it would indeed have been golden.

The nurse who conducts the clinic (there is no doctor) has almost no medicine. She is only 17—same age as the mother—with a year-and-a-half of elemental training. Three times a week she holds a clinic at Kyoe Waing and, other days, across the Salween river at a fall-back camp to which these people will go in case of attack.

She does what she can. Anemia and malnutrition, for which she has no treatment, are common. It is taken for granted in this humid jungle country that almost everyone will have malaria.

As we move on to talk with others, Ka The Htoo and her baby wait for the nurse's attention. Wait for the medicines the nurse does not have to give.

The 500 refugees here and across the river at Pu Mya Lu are fortunate to have any medical care. There are a total of *three* doctors for the 3 million people who live in these 20,000 square miles the Rangoon government considers to be the Burmese province of Kawthoolei (Kaw-too-*lay*) and which those who live in it, mostly Karens, regard as a full-fledged though, so far, unrecognized nation. It's one of the world's longest, saddest and least noticed struggles for national independence—or at least, autonomy—with grievances that make King George III look like America's benefactor.

Why were the 20 villagers killed? "No specific reason," Phy Ler Say tells me. Formerly an officer in the Burmese Forest Service, he is assistant chairman of the newly-organized Karen Christian Relief Committee. He and his wife speak the meticulous English one would expect to hear at Oxford. He is our translator.

"The Burmese think they have to subdue every village they can reach, because they believe all are in league with the independence movement," he explains. This region close to the Moei and Salween rivers—which form Kawthoolei's boundary with Thailand—is comparatively secure from attack; the last was eight years ago. The closer to the western border, however, the more vulnerable are the villages.

I did not propose to fight anybody's war. But I had to understand why hundreds of refugees had walked for days over tortuous mountain trails to this valley of the rivers, and why hundreds more, even thousands, might come.

Two men from the village of Mai Wei, about 100 miles away, tell me why they left their homes. Thaw Maw, a Karen, says, "The Burmese soldiers came and tied up people. There were beatings. We had 200 men in the village. Nine were killed."

Nga Tain, a Shan, adds, "While a mother was feeding her baby, soldiers took the woman out and raped her."

After the initial attack, the soldiers left. During the lull, 10 families made their escape. The next day the troops returned, encircling the village to prevent any from leaving, but these families in the camp had already gone. After seven days of walking, they arrived here.

"It was a major attack," says Nga Tain. "They came in three prongs, about a thousand of them altogether."

Lah Pwe tells how it was at his village near Mai Wei. The troops came often, usually at night, from their base which was just seven miles away. When this attack was launched before dawn, the villagers were alerted by watchmen.

"Often when the soldiers came, we took rice and hid in the jungle until they left," he tells me. "This time some of us decided to come here. We have heard that our village was burned."

Lah Pwe admits there had been provocation. Karen guerrillas had attacked the army post. The Burmese said it was the nearby villagers. They deny this, but do affirm their sympathy for the rebel cause. The villagers want to go home, but they believe the Burmese will not leave until (and if) they can be forced out by the Karen National Liberation Army (KNLA).

"Our land there is good land," says Thaw Maw.

That is more than can be said for the rugged terrain here along the Salween. However, in its ruggedness lies its comparative security. The guerrillas do not have the resources to launch a strong offensive. The Burmese cannot logistically support an attack into the mountains where upthrusting peaks rise almost vertically.

It is a stand-off war.

Karens have never trusted the Burmese who, generations ago, pushed them from their fertile lowlands into the inhospitable hills. During World War II, the Burmese took the side of the invading Japanese (until it was clear they were worse masters than the British). The Karens stayed loyal to the British and, with the Kachins and other hill peoples, sheltered downed Allied airmen who crashed while flying "the Hump" into China, often at the cost of their own lives.

After the war, when Burma received independence from Great Britain, the Karens pressed hard for their own independence but settled for the promise of autonomy within a union of states—a pledge that was never honored by the Burmese government. Kawthoolei sent two of its presidents to the negotiating table and both were murdered. There have been no negotiations since 1963.

Christians have an important stake in what happens in those hills, for we have many brothers and sisters there. When the gospel was introduced in 1877 by Adoniram and Ann Judson, American Baptist missionaries, the tribespeople of Burma were the most responsive. At the centennial celebration held by the Kachin Baptist Convention at Myitkyina, near the Chinese border, 73,000 people registered and more than 6,000 new converts were baptized.

Hundreds of missionaries from the denomination

served heroically until all foreign missionaries were forced out by the Rangoon government in 1966. Since then, American Baptists have given as much assistance to the church as possible. However, travel restrictions imposed by Rangoon make travel by foreigners into the tribal areas impossible through normal channels.

Estimates of Christians among all the Karens range from 10 to 15 percent. Buddhists and animists make up most of the rest. Leaders of the independence movement claim there are 6 million Karens in all of Burma—with half of them living in Kawthoolei. But the Burmese, primarily Buddhist, admit to only 1 million since they do not count as Karens those who adhere to Buddhism.

"What about that saffron-robed priest I saw in the refugee village?" I asked Mr. Ler Say.

"He was mistreated by the Burmese soldiers, which is why he came here," he said. "They do not respect even their own Buddhist priests, if they are Karens."

In fairness, it must be said that not all Karens support the independence movement, but even among those who have made their peace with Rangoon, most are sympathetic to the idea of a free or autonomous Karen state.

As we scramble back down to the river from the sloping plateau where Kyoe Waing was built four months ago—and where houses are still being put up for newcomers who live in makeshift quarters as they arrive—it is not hard to see the problems. The path leads along ridges between ingeniously terraced paddy fields, now rock-hard and barren, waiting the healing rains.

While sliding down the last bank to the beach and then struggling through the deep, loose sand to our waiting "longtailed" canoes—the kind needed to navigate the swift, shallow water of the dry season—I see something that makes my heart glad. We have not come to our brothers empty-handed. Stacked on a bamboo platform near the water's edge is Kyoe Waing's share of rice—300 sacks. Each sack holds 100 kilograms—220 pounds. The supply will last four months, and then the new crop will be coming in, if all goes well.

All does not invariably go well. Last year, at Pu Mya Lu across the river, they planted 16 tons of paddy seed and got only 30 baskets of rice! At the critical time, three days of needed soaking rains did not come, and there was no crop. On the riverbank there, too, sacks of rice await distribution. They are unguarded and undisturbed, though out of sight of the village, for there is no stealing in Kawthoolei. It couldn't happen in any Western country. But out here, where people are adjudged to be culturally underprivileged and even primitive, there is scrupulous honesty. There are no locks. No doors on houses, either, for that matter.

Mr. Ler Say tells me something else about these people who live temptingly near the notorious "Golden Triangle," that area where Burma, Thailand and China meet and where a major part of the world's opium is grown and then refined into heroin. He says: "In Kawthoolei, we have no drugs, no alcohol. And no Communism."

That cannot be said about the rest of Burma, which has its own home-grown Burmese Communist Party.

General Saw Bo Mya, commander of the KNLA and president of the Karen National Union (KNU), had told me how he rebuffed Communist offers of military assistance. He said that "when some of our own people left us to join the Communists in fighting the Rangoon government, we fought both them and the Burmese for three years. Then they came back to us."

He said firmly: "The work of Communists is the work of Satan."

Here is one border the free world won't have to worry about, I thought. That is, if the Karens can hold out long enough. Without help from some source, however, that is by no means a certainty.

Having arrived at Pu Mya Lu, we claw our way up a steep path to the house of Joshua Ler Say, director of this camp and our translator's son. Slipping off our shoes, we climb the ladder to an immaculate bamboo dwelling, open to the air for coolness, sun-drenched but with welcome shade. There is the immediate sense of family, of Christian companionship. Here are our brothers and sisters, living precariously but with a holy joy and confidence that fortifies my own soul.

We talk at length after lunch. I learn of the Karen seminary at Law Bwe Deh, 25 miles (40 kilometers) distant. Bombed out of its previous location at Papun, the school was moved to the more secure site two years ago, with five students. Now there are eight students pursuing the three-year course required before ordination. One year of practical evangelism is also a preordination requirement.

Pastor Robert Htwe, chairman of the Relief Committee, who has been with us all morning, shakes his head. It seems the future of the seminary is uncertain. Rice is in short supply and there is nothing to pay the four teachers.

"What would it take to keep it going?" I ask.

Pastor Robert ponders: "It would take a lot. As much as $750."

I dare not let my face register my gentle amusement. For a man who gets no salary, that is a large amount. But to me it seems so little, especially when I remember that the evangelists being trained are going into an area that is more receptive to the gospel than a hundred other nations.

"We will provide rice for the students and subsidy for the teachers," I promise. "But I think your figure isn't large enough. Let's make it $2,000, spread over two years."

The pastor's face glows as Mr. Ler Say puts it into

Karen. Even unexpressed, his joy was apparent.

Evangelists need tools, so we also agreed to provide slide projectors with small one-half kilowatt generators and sets of Bible slides. Pastor Robert says quietly, "With that, 20 percent of the people we reach would accept Christ."

Back at Atoo Wahy Lu, the village on the Moei River where General Bo Mya lives, Pi Pi Emma had earlier given us a clue to the openness of Karens to the gospel. (*Pi Pi* means "grandmother.") Emma Pawin, 77, is a kind of elder stateswoman, principal of the Central State High School, adviser to the KNU. Her sharp mind crackles. She loves young people and she loves the borning nation to which she has committed herself. If George Washington was the father of his country, Pi Pi Emma is the grandmother of hers.

She told me the remarkable folktale Karens have handed down from generation to generation. God gave a Golden Book and a Silver Book to his Burmese and Karen sons, the story goes, and a "Father" Book, or God Book, to a younger white brother. Someday, the ancestors said, the younger son would bring the God Book to his brothers.

When white missionaries came, the people were expecting them.

"There is even a song about it," Pi Pi Emma said. "God asked the Karen brother to go on a mission for him, but the Karen said he was too busy. He asked the Burmese brother to go, but he also said he was too busy. Then he asked the white brother, who answered, 'Yes, I will go.'"

There is a remarkable receptivity to the gospel in Kawthoolei, readied generations ago, perhaps by God Himself. And there is an inescapable message in Pi Pi Emma's song—a message for us.

Along a path that would have challenged a mountain goat, we walk to the church at Pu Mya Lu, where I had been asked to preach. There are 119 people in this village and it looks as if they are all in church (at 2:00 on a Monday afternoon!), with most of them in one of the two choirs. The floor is of dirt, the benches are built on posts driven into the ground, a plank in front of each for a desk, as the church also serves as the school.

Split bamboo—it's used for everything from building materials to toothpicks—extends part way up the sides to form the walls. On a bamboo platform at one end stands a table covered by an embroidered white cloth. Behind the table are four chairs, and I am directed to one; Mr. and Mrs. Ler Say and General Bo Mya take the others. A children's choir sings in carefully-learned English, "Welcome to you!" and I smile back. But when an adult choir swings into what is clearly a favorite of theirs, my eyes mist. They are singing in Karen, but I know the tune. As they sing, my lips form the words: *"Count your many blessings, name them one by one. Count your many blessings, see what God hath done."*

What blessings? How can these humble Christians who have so little of anything find blessings not only to count but to sing about? I am afraid my voice is not steady as I rise to speak, with Mrs. Ler Say interpreting.

Before I bring the Word, I say something like this: "Jesus knows everything you have suffered. He knows about your families you left behind. He knows about the tears you have shed. I have been in many refugee camps around the world. My only comfort is that Jesus is there with His people. In His own time He will deliver them. He said, 'I will never leave you nor forsake you.' Keep faith and hope alive in your hearts—"

The general speaks brief words of encouragement: "If we want victory"—and now Mrs. Ler Say is translating in reverse—"we must please God. We must be brave, for bravery will lead us to victory. May God bless you all."

I have not heard any generals speak like that, but I am not surprised. General Bo Mya had revealed himself in conversation, testimony and action to be a committed Christian.

"Even if other countries don't help us, we believe that God will help us," the general had told me. After he had distinguished himself as a young corporal, a British missionary chaplain had recommended him for a field promotion to captain on the spot. The stars of a general came in natural progression. When that missionary was expelled from Burma after independence, he returned secretly to live and die in Kawthoolei. There he was buried by loving Karen hands.

Bo Mya, a general since 1963, is a Seventh-Day Adventist. He attends not only two Adventist services on Saturday, but three Baptist services on Sunday. Pastor Robert Htwe conducts all five services. In addition, every household in Atoo Wahy Lu, including the general's own, holds evening family worship seven days a week.

His men speak of him not only with respect, but love. Major Wah Hin, commissary officer, who was at the general's home during our visit but at other times runs a trading post upriver at Mei Ta Waw, invariably refers to him as "my general."

"My general sent my son to a hospital in a neighboring country to have his arms operated on." Then he told me the story. When Major Wah Hin left to join the KNLA, the son had stayed behind in Burma with the rest of his family so the children could be in school. The separation lasted 12 years. "You have to sacrifice," said the major.

During that time, the young man was arrested by the Burmese who thought he could tell them where General Bo Mya kept his weapons and ammunition. Tying his hands behind his back, they hoisted him by the rope so that only his toes touched the ground. The next night they did the same. The third night, after a few hours, his arms pulled from their sockets. The next night, it took only an hour to dislocate them, and so it went for weeks. He was in prison for three-and-a-half years and came out with his arms horribly damaged. If he moved unexpectedly in his sleep, his arms came out of joint.

Upon his release, he joined his father and that's when "my general" sent him for the operation. At Mei Ta Waw, he took off his shirt so that I could see the scars on his shoulders. But I could not see the scars on his soul.

The Karens do not make prisoners of any Burmese soldiers they capture. They take their weapons and uniforms, then give them civilian clothes, feed them and show them kindness, talk to them about Karen desires for independence, ask them not to fight anymore and send them home to their families.

No one at any level of government in Kawthoolei—from president to school teachers to troops—receives a salary. Each is given a weekly ration of rice, depending on the size of his family. When the government comes by any money—usually from customs duties on consumer goods passing through Kawthoolei to Rangoon—it is shared equally, general down. Says Bo Mya, as if it explains everything, "The Burmese soldiers fight because they are paid."

The three doctors of Kawthoolei are based at a small "hospital" in Atoo Wahy Lu. When I ask Dr. Kho Taw, officer-in-charge, what instruments he has to work with, he is embarrassed to answer. "Two scalpels. Two pairs of retractors. Eight hemostats," he says.

"That is *all?*"

That is all.

No equipment for administering general anesthetic. No

way to do amputations or, for that matter, any surgery. The serious cases have to go to Thailand at great expense and over a bone-jarring stretch of road that would finish off anyone already half dead.

The small hospital itself is clean and airy. The "operating room" smells of disinfectant and has linoleum on the floor. A wooden table stands in the center.

We journey down the Salween to Me Leh Hte, a traditional animist village. These people are not refugees, but they are just as hungry. They simply cannot grow enough for their needs because of the rough terrain and the uncertain weather. My questions reveal they don't know much about growing vegetables. Rice is the basic crop, plus jungle fruit, coconut, durian and bananas. There are a few chickens for eating after they have been sacrificed to the spirits—enough to have meat maybe once a month. Pork? Once a year. The average annual family income is $50 to $75.

The child mortality rate is well over 50 percent. Some parents have only one or two children surviving—out of 10 born to them.

Against that background, I put a question: "What do you want most?"

"Food!" Several gave the same answer.

At this, a young man spoke up: "Food is not enough. Freedom is important. We need security to work."

The general is with us; these are his people, too, as are the refugees. He makes a wry observation: "The main problem is health. They are not physically able to do hard labor."

But these people are so busy growing rice—rather, *trying* to grow it—that they are not able to do anything else. If they were healthy enough and knew how to do it, they could produce an adequate supply of rice plus a few cash crops. But the land must be cleared and since the jungle grows right down to the river, that is back-breaking work. Such a Western commonplace as a gasoline-driven chainsaw would open up a whole new level of possibilities.

All of which emphasizes how impossible it is to separate needs. They are all intertwined. Nor can the physical ministry and the gospel-telling be separated.

"What do you think happens to a person when he dies?" I ask the elders of the village of Me Leh Hte. They have the feeling they are different from animals. Some believe they will be "somewhere," but others think there is nothing beyond. Some are too weary to care.

"What have you heard about Jesus?" I query. The story is not very clear to them. They don't understand what it's all about. A few have become Christians, but animistic beliefs prevail.

I note the contrast between the people here—clothing and bodies unwashed, despite the plentiful supply of clean water in the nearby river—and those at the predominantly Christian village. Although the population is over a thousand in this cluster of villages, there are only two schools, one teacher in each, 17 pupils in one and 15 in the other. It may be motivation. More likely, these people are just too sick, too lacking in energy, to do more than survive.

They are not refugees, except from hunger; they have lived and starved here for generations. It is in villages like these that Pastor Robert sees his 20 percent increase in converts.

After four days, leaving General Bo Mya, Major Wah Hin, Pastor Robert Htwe and all our other friends, is like leaving a long-lost, new-found family. As we wave good-bye, I think of travelers on another road who said out of their richness of blessing what I was feeling: *"Did not our hearts burn within us?"* For it had been as I had said in that service in the little bamboo church high above the Salween: "We have come that we might be encouraged by each other." And Mrs. Ler Say had replied, "Because of this visit, we know that someone loves us."

Kawthoolei. Here where every name means something, this one means, "Land full of peace and riches."

Not yet, Lord, but maybe with your blessing and some help from friends—

4

Sustaining a Fragile Hope

Philippines

Everything seemed wrong.

The time. The place. The subject.

And me.

Most of all, me. What did I know about life-and-death issues of the tribal Batac people of the Philippines? I had been among them only a few hours and yet I found myself involved in a tense, dramatic conversation between a young husband and wife.

They seemed scarcely aware of my presence as they debated one of the most crucial issues that a husband and wife can ever face—whether or not they could afford to have another baby already on the way.

Dominga is nursing curly-headed, seven-month-old Elizabeth as she talks with her husband, Primitivo. She is pregnant again and Primitivo wants her to drink the "bitter root" and abort the fetus now growing inside her. This is not a detached philosophical conversation, but a question of raw survival. It is not taking place in a doctor's antiseptic office or the counseling room of a social worker. We are on the remote island of Palawan, sitting cross-legged on the slatted bamboo floor of an open-walled, one-room hut. The hut, resting slightly askew on its stilts, holds no possessions, but it is the couple's home.

We are talking about the hard life of the Batac tribespeople on the primitive island on the west side of the Filipino archipelago. They tell me that half of the children born to Batac mothers die before they are seven years old. This is what concerns Primitivo. The couple had watched their firstborn, a son, die just two days short of his first birthday.

Primitivo is afraid the same thing will happen to Elizabeth. The problem is food. There simply is not enough of it for another mouth. I could see that even now Elizabeth's eyes were taking on that glassy look which indicates—at the very least—severe vitamin A deficiency that can cause blindness.

The third baby is coming too soon. Primitivo is overwhelmed by his looming responsibility. The couple knows nothing about modern birth control and family planning. Families are planned by drinking the root brew that keeps the babies from coming too close together.

Dominga finally agrees to follow the tribal traditions and her husband's wishes. She will drink what a pregnant woman drinks when she doesn't want the baby. But for all her anguish, Dominga—the twice-over mother—is scarcely able to make a woman's decision.

She is only 13 years old.

I also am in anguish, but for this child/mother, because human wisdom fails me in this situation. I promise to pray that God may guide them in their decision. They nod, but I know that their concept of God is still very imperfect and that the decision will ultimately be based on economics and daily realities, not on some kind of vague spiritual guidance.

But before I can begin to word a prayer, Dominga's

mother, Pacita, comes by and her bare feet nimbly bring her up the four-foot ladder into the "house." She proves to be a lively conversationalist.

Pacita had heard the last snatches of our conversation, so she enters the dialogue with her daughter and son-in-law. Dominga is the oldest of her two surviving children—six others died. Pacita's concern is also intense. The lives of her grandchildren, and possibly her daughter, hang in the balance. She says that if she could, she would take Elizabeth and raise her so that Dominga could have the other child.

The offer causes animated discussion among the three. My interpreter keeps me informed. It is pointed out that Pacita has her own eight-year-old daughter. Food is also a problem for her. She agrees that she couldn't do it without financial help. That stops the conversation, but the impossible dream had for a moment given a glimmer of hope.

I enter the conversation. How much help would Pacita need? A big can of powdered milk each month and some bottles. Anything else? Some vitamins. That's all? Probably.

Now over to Primitivo, who's been listening. Would he agree to the arrangement if I can make it possible for his little Elizabeth to grow up healthy? His stern look dissolves. Pacita grins with delight over the prospect of having a tiny one to love. Dominga is as happy as a little girl with a new doll, which is exactly what she reminds me of as she rocks Elizabeth gently on her lap.

The crisis is over. At least one life has been saved. Probably two. The jungle will not claim this unborn Batac baby.

As the conversation became more relaxed, Pacita told me about the exploitation of the Batacs, a small and peaceful tribe, which goes all the way back to Spanish explorers.

The leaders of these short-statured, dark-skinned people feared that, with only 3,000 remaining, they would disappear from the earth. The Batacs are one of 41 identifiable aboriginal tribes in the Philippines, totalling 4 million people. The government calls them "tribal minorities" and tries to protect them with whatever laws it can pass and enforce. But many tribal groups, such as the Batacs, have no written language and not even the rudiments of an education that would allow them to claim their rights.

All of the living Batacs are found on Palawan, one of the largest and most primitive of the more than 7,000 Philippine islands, only half of which even have names. The province of Palawan alone has 1769 islets, and there is only one city, Puerto Princesa. The provincial population is about 365,000, with nearly one-fourth that number being cultural minorities.

The Batacs, especially, have had a hard existence. Pushed higher and higher into the mountains by the lowlanders—sometimes by sheer pressure, sometimes by being cheated out of their tribal lands—they have been left with the most inaccessible, rugged terrain on which to scratch out an existence.

They have tried to farm the sharply-angled landscape, using the slash-and-burn technique and a form of dry gardening called *kaingin,* but with negligible success. It seems that both nature and man have conspired against the gentle clan. Since 70 percent of Palawan is primeval forest, it is very desirable to logging interests who, under government contract, prohibited the Batacs from going into their own ancestral lands. Then the government itself made it impossible, as a conservation measure, for anyone to gather honey or hunt wild animals without a permit. These were two principal elements in the Batac diet, but among a totally illiterate people no one knew how to acquire a permit.

Facing these problems in the mountains and squeezed by the incursion of the lowlanders into their rice-growing lands, the Batacs began to turn inward and participate in their own unplanned genocide. Intermarriage within close families resulted in weak genes while malnutrition and disease contributed to a high death rate.

It was in that kind of setting that we found 36 families living in a secluded valley in the mountains above Roxas, a community on the northeast coast, which has a dirt airstrip, silica mines and not much else. A year of periodic contact passed before the people were trusting enough to think about moving out of their valley of misery onto some productive land below their mountain which was made available to them.

The reservation set aside by the government and purchased by private funds consists of almost 500 acres of good rice land which can be irrigated. While the acquisition went on, 12 families moved down and cleared a significant area for farming. The plan is to eventually bring 200 families out of the mountains and make it possible for each of them to own the land they farm.

I talked with several men who gathered at the well. "It is better here than in the mountains," says 75-year-old Emilio Tugnaw, the oldest man in the barrio. "Since I was a small boy, until now, life has been difficult. On many days I would eat only once. Sometimes I went to sleep without anything to eat."

Heads nodded as the old patriarch spoke of the experience of them all. Finally, they had been reduced to eating land turtles, which themselves had become scarce.

Now the people do eat, at least most of the time. But even the new land is something less than the Garden of Eden. For instance, farming is next to impossible without good work animals. In this region of tropical rainfall, two indigenous weeds—cogon grass and hagony—quickly

take over the land unless you keep it under constant cultivation. That means plowing the soil deep by means of a
carabao, the Filipino version of the water buffalo. And that
is another impossibility without outside help, for a carabao
costs $300, far beyond the ability of a Batac to own one in
a lifetime.

Then there's the matter of a school. There is no education in the whole village. Not a single adult in the tribe has
ever gone to school. I raise the matter as we sit in the
shade for a long discussion of their problems. I put the
question through an interpreter: "Would you like to have
school?" A murmur went through the crowd, and even
some hands shot up quickly in a unanimous "Yes!"

"We hope that our children can go to school and serve
as the light to us," said Don Fernando, one of the barrio
leaders. Now they are afraid to send their children to the
lowland school, because the Batac children look and dress
differently and have been teased and bullied by the other
children.

Moises, the other co-captain in the barrio, says they
want education for the adults, too—enough to keep from
being cheated, enough to be able to get what they need at
fair prices instead of the higher costs charged the tribal
minorities by unscrupulous merchants. They want to be
able to sell sweet potatoes for the 5 or 10 pesos they
should get instead of the one peso they are paid. And they
want to be able to read the Bible and write.

The government will put in a school if the people can
get the land declared a tribal reservation and if there are
enough children to attend. The magic number is at least 20
families—that would mean a potential of 40 to 80 students, except that the Batacs have fewer children, so
more families need to be coaxed from their mountain
seclusion.

That is not easy with the present tensions existing

between the tribal people and the lowlanders. A project director tells how it is: "Pastor Bundac from Roxas comes in and out on his motorcycle. He has been told by the lowlanders to stop or his life will be in danger. But he comes anyway. We're trying to establish good feelings with the lowlanders. When you are dealing with minorities, you can't just jump into the mountains and help them. You've got to help the people along the trail."

The lowlanders, not unlike some people from my part of the world, think that dirt and hardship is the normal lot of minorities. They argue that if God had not wanted them to be uneducated and have a high death rate, He would have put them in some other place.

The lowlanders also feel an economic threat as the minorities start back down the mountains. Formerly, the lowlander took the land he wanted because he was better educated, had carabaos and even weapons. The threat of having that privileged status come to an end upsets many of them.

At the new village site, the first improvement was a well with a hand pump so that clean water would be available. The people are beginning to catch on to hygiene and simple health procedures. They have built their first communal outdoor toilet, ingeniously constructed of bamboo and bark sheets. This is an important addition to barrio life because the deworming process has begun—one girl was found to have 21—and sanitation will help prevent reinfection.

The Batacs still have a lot to learn about the relationship between dirt and disease, but they are learning fast. One item that we carried in our Toyota jeep was there by special request—a bright red dishpan-size plastic tub. Since Don Fernando had requested it, he carries it from the jeep triumphantly. He is a man of about 40, under five feet tall and clad only in a pair of shorts and friendly smile.

"Bring us a tub and we will take baths," he had said. Appropriately, the tub arrived in time for Saturday night! Baths until now have been purely accidental, as when crossing streams or getting caught in a downpour.

Primitivo had earlier indicated a desire to bathe also, but he explained that he had only one pair of pants, and if he washes them he has nothing else to wear. He says he would bathe every day and wash and change his clothes, if he could afford to buy soap and clothes.

He is not exaggerating or begging. It is a fact. Now every centavo—and there are only a few of those—must go for food for Elizabeth and the pregnant Dominga. Primitivo works for the lowlanders when he can. He owns no land. "If I just had two boxes!" he exclaims, both in hope and frustration. (One "box" of land is about 100 square feet.)

When the lowlanders want him for a day's work, he is paid about five pesos, roughly 75 cents. He is heavily in debt. Like other Batacs, he acquired his wife by paying a price to her parents. Dominga cost him 30 pesos, but he hasn't been able in three years to go beyond the down payment of five pesos! When he finishes paying what is still due, he will have full rights to his wife that will stand up in any court. Then if another man ever wants his wife and Dominga wants to leave him, by tribal custom the other man would have to pay Primitivo double, or 60 pesos.

"If I work hard, and if things are better, I think I can pay off the bride price in a year," he says. A year of the hardest kind of labor to pay off a debt of $4.50!

Pastor Bundac confirms this is not unusual among the Batacs. They have been brought to absolute poverty by a civilized world that has no room for a people who have become a cultural anachronism.

This man who rides his motorcycle out to bring spiritual knowledge to the Batacs in spite of threats by his fellow lowlanders told me that he was challenged back in 1966 to take the gospel to this tribal minority by a missionary who was leaving the area. He felt a burden for the people and tried to do it.

"But," he said, "every time I went up there to preach to them they told me how hungry they were, how poor they were, and how many needs they had."

Tears sprang to his eyes even now as he recalled, "They asked me if there wasn't some way I could help them. I never had anything to offer them and it finally got so that I just quit going. I couldn't preach to them empty-handed. Then in 1977 a Christian relief agency put help in my hands."

For 11 years there was no gospel witness among these Batacs simply because this pastor, who was ready and willing, was not able to take both word and deed, witness and service, to a waiting people. Now that he has material assistance to offer them along with the gospel, Pastor Bundac plans to start twice-weekly Bible studies.

"The Batacs are very open to the gospel," he said, and my own questioning of their beliefs confirmed this.

They even built a road so that we could drive all the way to the river at the edge of their village instead of having to trek the last few hundred yards. It was a project of immense proportions—and worthy, I think, of the name "Batac Freeway" which we bestowed upon it—considering that sizable trees and heavy vegetation had been removed with nothing more than bolo knives.

The people were there again to see us off at the end of the day. With great nimbleness, they crossed the bridge they had built; we edged our way across the round, widely-spaced logs that could easily have turned an ankle or worse.

They had given us the best they had to offer—the hospitality of their shade, a glass filled with coffee which we shared around, and their beautifully simple friendship.

As we drove back over the "Batac Freeway," I remembered the words of Pacita, "We consider you our father."

Small wonder, then, that I kept waving until our jeep turned into the dirt trail and the village disappeared from sight. Isn't that what *you* do when you say good-bye to your children?

5

Where Have All the Nomads Gone?

Horn of Africa

The hot desert winds whipped up spectacular dust devils that reached high into the sky as they danced over the sere and barren landscape.

Stretched out in front of me was a desert country occupied only by graves. No flowers. No whitewashed grave markers. No carved epitaphs. Just rows and rows of graves, each covered with a layer of heavy stones to protect the body beneath from scavenging animals. Scrawny thorn bushes gave the whole scene a surreal look.

But I had only to turn and look behind me at the bustling activity in Agabar camp to return to the world of reality. I was in the African country of Somalia in the middle of one of the world's worst refugee problems.

My colleagues and I had walked directly from the Agabar camp hospital (too grand a name, really, for a collection of three tents) to the camp cemetery. In retrospect, that seems to have been the right order of events. That's the way it had happened for so many who lay in those shallow graves—except that they had been carried there by the gentle hands of relatives.

No one knows how many people have been buried there during the 18 months the camp has been in existence, but camp officials told me 700 children died during the first three months alone.

Now Agabar, population 42,000, has been closed to newcomers for some time, and those refugees who continue to stream across the border from Ethiopia— estimated then at about a thousand a day—are sent to new camps, many of them located near Agabar around the northern Somalia city of Hargeisa.

One of these new camps is Saba'at. But after being opened in November, 1979, Saba'at was declared closed to new arrivals four months later when the population reached 58,000.

Then the cycle started over again. And the end, I was told, is nowhere in sight. Sayeed Gase, national refugee commissioner, told me over tea that his government estimated the total number of refugees at nearly 1½ million, with more than half that number living outside the camps among the local population in all kinds of desperate circumstances.

Actually, those in the camps are only a little better off than those outside. Because of national poverty, the assistance the government can give is minimal. And the growing international aid involvement is also minimal and not increasing fast enough to keep abreast of Somalia's burgeoning need.

As the problem mushroomed out of all manageable proportions, it had remained virtually hidden from the rest of mankind. Somalia is not, after all, at the crossroads of the world. The refugees themselves had gathered on generous pieces of desert far away from towns. A trip to visit them can range from inconvenient to arduous. It is small wonder that this largest concentration of refugees had remained at the bottom of the list of neglected ones.

Who are these people and why are they running?

In order to understand the problem, some background is necessary. Located in East Africa on what is called the Horn of Africa, Somalia is one of the poorest nations on the continent. Annual per capita income is estimated at about $100. The population numbers between 4-5 million, of which some 1 million follow a nomadic way of life while another million-and-a-half are seminomadic.

Since migration is a way of life for Somalis, they have always treated with disdain the country's international boundaries, which were drawn by colonial powers seemingly more interested in extricating themselves from their restless colonies than in preserving ethnic solidarity within them.

Thus ethnic Somalis are found in both Somalia and Ethiopia. On the west, Somalia has its longest border with Ethiopia—over 1,000 miles, and it is here the problem has arisen. Ethiopia's Ogaden Desert area is populated mostly by nomadic or a few sedentary Somali-speaking groups or other tribes not related to the dominant Amharic ruling class of Ethiopia. It is from the Ogaden that the refugees come.

I stopped to talk at one Somali hut in Saba'at to try to get an accurate picture of what is happening to the fleeing nomads. Five people were living in the small hut, called an *agal,* constructed from bent limbs of desert trees and covered with pieces of woven straw and grass. Halimo Ahmed, the 50-year-old woman who was head of this household, talked to me with great animation through the small doorway. In the hut were her daughter and the daughter's three children, the youngest of whom was just 10 days old. Halimo spoke firmly, vigorously, dramatically. She was typical of most Somalis I met; they are an attractive and dynamic people, easy to relate to and uninhibited in conversation with foreigners.

She was proud of her new granddaughter whom they had named Fadumo. When I asked Halimo about her own husband, her face became sad and her voice softened. Her hands moved rhythmically as if to orchestrate her words. He was killed in 1977. "Shot," she said, "by the enemy." Halimo said she then went to live with her daughter and son-in-law.

As she continued, her voice became high-pitched and agitated. Her gestures no longer flowed; now her hands began to chop the air.

"The Cubans came with the Ethiopians," she told me, "and burned down our house. That is why we had to leave. They shot our animals just like they have killed our strong young people. We have no food, no shelter, no clothing, and the enemy has taken our property."

Her son-in-law stayed behind to become a "freedom fighter." With everything taken away, Halimo, her pregnant daughter and the two children started walking toward Somalia. They were four days on the road, sleeping out at night, when they were picked up by a truck belonging to the Western Somalia Liberation Front (WSLF). It took them six more days to reach the border. They had now been at Saba'at Camp for five months. Her son-in-law did not know where the family was. He knew only that they left for safety in Somalia.

Approximately 90 percent of those in the camps are women, children and old people. Like Halimo's son-in-law, most of the young men and fathers have stayed behind and joined the WSLF. Although they are outnumbered and outgunned, the ragtag army has managed to occupy tens of thousands of Ethiopian soldiers and their Cuban advisers. In fact, for a brief period during 1977-78, with the help of their kinsmen from Somalia, these fighters wrested the Ogaden from Ethiopian control.

However, with massive Russian and Cuban support,

the Ethiopians have reestablished their authority over the main towns in the region. Apparently they are now trying to secure the area by clearing the Ogaden of its indigenous Somali population. It has meant the dislocation of perhaps 2 million people.

The heart-wrenching scenes I saw at the camp are still with me. As we walked around, people came from everywhere bringing their sick and malnourished children. One father brought his five-year-old son in his arms. The child was recovering from measles, but now had an extreme case of diarrhea. The boy was so weak, he could not hold up his head. There were no medicines in the camp and I had none to give him.

I cried when the father turned and walked sadly away. And just as I turned to go down to the dry riverbed where people were digging for water, a mother approached begging me to help her two-year-old daughter who was so malnourished that the child was little more than skin and bones.

Again, all I could do was tell the mother that a supplemental feeding program for the children was due to begin soon. The next day we bought powdered milk on the local market in Hargeisa so that special feeding for the worst cases could begin immediately.

An initial survey by a doctor showed that 30 percent of the children under five need "therapeutic feeding," indicating severe malnutrition, and another 40 percent need "supplementary feeding," indicating moderate malnutrition. Thus 70 percent of the children are suffering from varying degrees of malnutrition.

Another scene that is etched into my memory happened late in the afternoon of my last day in the camps. Our Land Rover crossed over a dry riverbed and began to climb toward the plateau which had been designated as the site of a new camp.

It was about 4:30 P.M. when we arrived. The chill night winds of the desert were just beginning to blow. Three old trucks pulled up just before we did, carrying several hundred people who had recently arrived at the border. As in every instance, they were all either old people or women with young children.

I watched the refugees as they climbed down after their long ride. This was their new "home," though there was nothing here but scraggly thorn bushes and stones. Most of them seemed too numb and tired to do anything more than walk a few steps away from the trucks and sit down. They carried only the most meager of possessions—usually one small bundle into which was tied everything they owned. A few produced dried animal skins that would protect them from the bare ground. Later, some gathered sticks and started small fires for boiling tea.

It was in the midst of this late afternoon scene that I met Ardo Abdullai. I had watched her walk away from the truck with her two small children—one a boy, about five years old, and the other a babe in arms. For all her weariness and hunger, she walked with a regal bearing, and a beauty shone out from her fatigued and grimy face.

As with all these mothers, I found her energetic, expressive and resilient. The baby girl she was holding was just four months old. She had left her home in Diredawa, she told me, a few weeks after the baby was born. "I wanted food and safety for my children," she said.

Her first husband and father of her son was killed in the fighting. Sometime later she had married his brother in order that her son might have a father. They had been blessed with a daughter, but she saw no future for her children in a land where there was fighting every day.

So she left and walked for two months to reach the border. Her husband stayed behind to fight, she said.

Then, with tears in her eyes, she told me, "I have heard that he was killed also."

We were both quiet for a little while.

I asked her what it felt like to be a widow twice, with two children, a refugee with no roof over her head tonight, and with a future as uncertain as the shifting desert sands. I was deeply touched by what she told me.

"Look at me. You can see that I have no clothes, no food, no shelter, no future. But I do not ask anything for myself. I ask only for my children. I hope from dear God that mothers everywhere will help us take care of our children."

I promised Mrs. Abdullai that I would tell all the mothers I could about her hopes and prayers for all the mothers and children who are homeless refugees in Somalia.

And I promised God that if He would make it possible, I would work night and day to see that those little ones don't end up in shallow desert graves, covered with a layer of stones to protect the bodies from wild animals that scavenge the sands at night.

6
Shattered People, Broken Lives

Lebanon

Some say there was two hours notice.

Others insist there was none.

In a camp of 60,000 it's not easy to get the word around, even when warning leaflets are dropped. Besides, it was not a camp as we think of the word. Ein-el-Hilweh was—and *was* is the right word—a congested city of concrete apartment buildings and block houses a kilometer east of Sidon. Begun 40 years ago for victims of an earthquake that hit this part of Lebanon, Ein-el-Hilweh took on a permanency and became, over the years, a growing haven for Palestinian refugees.

There is no Ein-el-Hilweh anymore. It died in 1982 under the bombs of Israel's invasion of Lebanon. The stench of its death was still in the air when I was there three weeks after the fateful night. Never before had I seen such total destruction. If the world's war-makers want to see what saturation bombing looks like, they should look here. Israel, the country skilled in making the desert blossom like a rose, knows also how to turn rose into desert.

Block after block of crumpled, tangled wreckage is all that is left. Plus an unknown number of bodies. There must be hundreds down there under the rubble—the permeating odor of decaying flesh tells you that much. Refugees who escaped say that as many as 8,000 died. The Red Cross puts the number at 1500. Either way, it's one of the major massacres of modern times.

"We will not bomb Ein-el-Hilweh if all the fighters come out," said the Israelis. However, the fighters of the Palestine Liberation Organization (PLO)—whatever their number was—stayed in. Presumably. And so the fire fell on the innocent, too, simply because they were in the way.

How do you evacuate a city in two hours, even if everyone is ready and desperate to leave? How do you empty a football stadium in minutes, even when there is no panic, no urgency beyond beating the next fan to the parking lot? I don't know the answer.

And for many refugees, there must come a point when, despairing of running, they run no more.

Some did get out. At a food distribution depot set up in a school in Sidon, I talked with a number of people who had lived in Ein-el-Hilweh. Full of what they had seen and been through, everyone wanted to talk.

Someone tells us that the first planes came at five o'clock in the evening; from just after midnight until eight the next evening the bombing was continuous. For three days the pounding went on. Everybody here has friends who died in the attack. A woman makes a chopping motion across the knees of a baby another woman is holding, saying she saw a baby at Ein-el-Hilweh who had both legs blown off.

Says 13-year-old Mahir, "I thought I would die. I was so scared." He says there is no water in the school where they have taken refuge, but they found a broken water main. Ten to 15 refugees live in each room of the school.

Zachyi, a 22-year-old mother of children ages 3, 1½ and 9 months, whose grace and inherent beauty are such she could have been cast for a Bible drama, apologizes for her filthy dress; it is the only one she has, she explains. She had to leave the school where they are now living at 4:30 this morning to get here at eight o'clock. She walked, she says. How else? Unless one has money, there is no other means of transportation and no other place to get food.

There are fewer refugees than usual here this Sunday morning, for the section many of them come from has been sealed off in one of the periodic and unpredictable Israeli searches for members of the Palestine Liberation Organization. The sweep method used is ironically reminiscent of Warsaw. Those caught in the net have to pass before masked informers who make a quick judgment: "PLO," "Not PLO." Some have been through this harrowing experience as many as five times.

In the courtyard at the food depot where names are being checked to make sure that today's distribution is equitable, four school desks cordon off an unexploded shell buried to almost its full length in the concrete.

An older woman, whose husband, Naif, is porter and watchman here at the center, invites us into the eight-by-eight foot room where three and sometimes five of the family sleep, cook, live. They are lucky; the room goes with Naif's job. We sit on the narrow couch and Naif's wife shows us snapshots of their children, including three sons captured by the Israelis 20 days ago. They were hauled off with their hands tied behind them. They are in a prison at Tyre, she thinks. She is worried about what will happen to them. The oldest, 23, is sick. The others are 16 and 17. A 14-year-old son lives here.

"How do you feel about the war?" I ask.

As she replies, her eyes fill. "Wars bring headaches

and tears and separation from the family." She fingers the snapshots of her missing sons, now her only tangible link, and her eyes overflow. "It is better to be dead than to live this way," she says, not with bitterness but with sadness.

The family home was originally in Haifa, she tells me. Refugees from Israel in 1948, they went to Tyre in southern Lebanon for three years, then to Sidon, where they have lived for 20 years in Ein-el-Hilweh.

We try to comfort her: "Your sons who were taken will return."

She responds wistfully, as if seeking assurance, "*Will* they return?" Again, tears flow as she says almost to herself, "They are sweet children."

When we have both recovered our composure, I ask her, "What do the Palestinian people want most of all?"

"We want our homes. Food and water. Vegetables. A normal life. Nothing great—just a normal life."

Daughter Kaltoum with two-month-old Rami comes into the crowded room. I ask Kaltoum what she wants Rami to be when he grows up. What will she reply? Liberator? Guerrilla fighter? General?

"A doctor," she says, as if she has said it many times.

"Do you really think that will happen?" I ask gently.

"If God provides, why not?"

Why not, indeed? And maybe a peacemaker besides, I think. Someone must do the healing.

Before we leave, Naif brings in a bowl of cherries he has hurriedly gone out to find. As he puts it down before us he speaks the traditional words of hospitality: "May your road in the future be full of light."

And may yours, is the response of my heart.

I ask if we can pray for the family and the missing boys, and Naif's wife responds with a world view that is at once a rebuke and a blessing: "All the people in the world deserve to have their place." My colleague prays in Arabic, and we leave, feeling a kinship that transcends religion and politics.

Across the street I come face to face with the gross horror of indiscriminate warfare. The place: Kineye School, Sidon, a Lebanese government secondary school for girls. Three weeks ago today it happened. No students were in the school, but during the afternoon, refugees arrived from Tyre, trying to keep ahead of the fighting. Hundreds of them, along with some of the local people, crowded into the lowest basement, seeking shelter from the bombing that was outracing them. The Israelis had urged them to get out of the way, and they had.

I visualized the scene. It is evening. Families are settling down in the darkness that comes early. Mothers are trying to comfort their crying, hungry children. Some have brought blankets; they are needed more to soften the hardness of the concrete floor for the little ones than as covering. As midnight nears, most of the children sleep. They have heard and felt the reverberations of shell and bomb and rocket before. The women cannot sleep until sheer exhaustion overtakes them. The men, unable to keep their families out of harm's way, feel frustrated, helpless. They cannot sleep.

Ein-el-Hilweh, not far away, is getting most of it. But Sidon proper does not escape. The building reels with each blast. The floor picks up concussions like a giant seismograph. The huddled refugees cringe, babies waken and cry. There is no sleep now for anyone.

Then at 2:30 in the morning, an aerial bomb slices into Kineye School. It rips bodies apart, strews arms and legs and pieces of what had been living, breathing human beings a second before. The concussion takes the rest.

No more running. No more crying. Now they sleep.

And here I am three weeks later where no observer is supposed to be, seeing what no observer is supposed to see. The bodies and pieces of bodies lie untouched, save for the lime that the local Red Cross has spread. That keeps down the smell of death somewhat. But Kineye School is a charnel house; body fluids, creeping across the basement floor from the stack of bodies, are ankle deep in places. It is possible to count 50 or so bodies. The rest are piled atop each other, hurled there by the blast that took their lives. We are told there are 255 altogether in the helter-skelter pile. It looks that high.

Later I asked, "Why doesn't someone bury them?"

Why, indeed does not "someone"? It would take trucks and bulldozers and heavy equipment. Only the Israelis have what it would take, and their army seems to have other things on its agenda, other uses for its bulldozers and half-tracks.

I come up out of the basement, shaken, gulping fresh air. An old woman who lives across the street comes out to see what we are doing. I ask her what happened. Still deeply affected, she jabbers in English and I make out, "Don't ask me. I have mind no more." Little wonder. We walk around the crater left by another bomb that fell between her house and the school. She is fortunate to be alive. Maybe.

There is traffic both ways on the road between Sidon and Beirut, made worse by the interminable waits at checkpoints where cars line up by the hundreds to be cleared or not. Some of the occupants hold green leaflets that have just been dropped, telling civilians to leave, but the leaflets don't seem to guarantee or expedite anyone's exit. Military traffic takes priority. The sheer magnitude of this one visible piece of the Israeli war machine is incredible. David seems determined to become Goliath. Perhaps someone in charge should reread the Bible story.

Meanwhile, back in Beirut the East and West sections are divided by what is called the "Green Line." The East is dominated by the rightist Christian forces, though here "Christian" carries more of a cultural than a religious connotation. The West is primarily Muslim; the PLO and other Muslim militia groups provide the military presence; here most of the Palestinians live. The bombing of West Beirut has caused some thousands to leave, but residents believe at least half a million remain.

Crossing the Green Line is an adventure in survival, no matter how many times one does it. Even youngsters on the West side can be seen carrying Kalashnikov automatic rifles; some dress in one kind of uniform or another, some not. To be cleared at one checkpoint does not mean you are home free; the fellow with the gun at the next one may be going by different rules.

I crossed the Green Line several times to be with Dennis Hilgendorf, a Lutheran who came in 1967 as a missionary and stayed to found the Contact and Resource Center (CRC). In prewar times, the CRC ministered to drug addicts and handicapped people. Today the staff helps victims of the war.

Dennis and his family live in an apartment building in a nice section of West Beirut called Roushi. A picture window opens onto a view of the Mediterranean. The view was especially clear on my first visit. Reason: no window. A few days before, a shell from an Israeli gunboat crashed through it, hurtling three feet over the head of Heather, age 8, and exploding in the wall behind which 3-year-old Nicholas was standing. Shattering glass fell all around Heidi, age 15, sitting in a chair, but left her untouched.

Phosphorus in the shell started fires at the front of the house. Acrid smoke filled the inside. Seconds later, another shell smashed into the outer wall, veered off and destroyed the elevator shaft next to the apartment. Two more landed upstairs, and two next door. By God's grace, no one was killed.

It is hard to imagine anyone getting out unscathed, physically or emotionally. Yet as soon as the children realized they were safe, the two older ones insisted on going upstairs to help their Muslim neighbors.

"How long do you plan to stay here on the West side?" I asked Dennis, when the cease-fire—negotiated the day after his home was shelled—became more tenuous by the moment and the Israelis were dropping more pamphlets warning people to get out while they could.

"We play it day by day," he said. "I'm not a hero. I have a family. For every crisis situation, I have developed my own contingency plans—and then I throw them away and stay. Now I'm doing it again. I will stay as long as I feel the Lord is calling me to a need here. If I become part of the problem rather than the solution because of hatred or impatience or lack of love or fear, that will be the time to leave. Right now, the Lord has given me the guidance to be here."

I'll dispute only one thing Dennis said. By anyone's measure but his own, he *is* a hero. And his rescue shop is not even a yard from hell. It is in the middle of it.

The story of Beirut is written primarily in the language of shattered people and broken lives. The story of the Rashida family is a typical example. When the father was killed in the bombing of Sidon, the oldest son fell apart emotionally. He managed to get himself on a boat, or maybe he went to Syria—nobody knows. He was the eldest, and it was his job to take care of the family, but it was too much for him.

The widow and remaining son came to Beirut where daughter Lelia is a student at the American University. Then the younger son was killed in one of the attacks on West Beirut. They didn't know he was missing until he was found dead on the street the morning after the attack. The mother, who has never recovered from the shock of her husband's death, was totally overwhelmed.

"That's just one of the thousands of families here in Beirut who simply haven't been able to face what has happened so quickly," Dennis says sadly.

Lelia, the 21-year-old Rashida daughter, is maturing emotionally and spiritually. She has become a member of one of the volunteer groups working with Dennis in refugee relief. Is Lelia, from a Muslim family, a Christian? She told Dennis, "I believe in a Lord who is beyond myself. He is One you and I are trying to get to know." She is surely not far from the kingdom; maybe she's closer than a lot of distant unscarred Christians would suppose.

I talked with refugees camped in Sanayeh Park on the West side of the Green Line. When one young Palestinian learned that I was an "Americani," he raced off to his little shelter and came back with an automatic rifle at the ready. Other Palestinians managed to talk him out of his obvious intention, explaining that although I was an American, I was there to help. Even if you are not looking down the barrel of a gun, it's an uncomfortable feeling to be an American in a Palestinian refugee camp. They dump on you all the feelings they have for Americans who supply the weapons that are destroying them.

A woman from Rashedieh camp, near Tyre, tells me that the first raid three weeks ago drove them to Beirut. The husband says that it was American bombs and American ammunition that leveled their home. "Tell America, please," he said, "to do something about it."

A woman named Suraiya says to my son Eric, "You are taking pictures of me here, and I come from a nice house. This is not the way I want to live." Her family came from the Chouf district, a Druze settlement, in the mountains east of the Beirut airport where shelling had been intense. They stayed at the City Sportif, a sports stadium, the first place in Beirut to be bombed. Then they moved here to the park. Uprooted, bereaved, her despair overflowed.

"The bombs came and now we have nothing," she says, weeping. Like the woman in Sidon yesterday, she brings out pictures of her family to show me. Everyone has pictures, if little else. She had 20 people in her extended family, but five died in the first attack at Chouf. The only food I can see is some chick-pea paste (a staple in Lebanon), half an onion, a jar with a few olives, and a little flour.

She puts her hand to her heart when we shake hands in parting.

Mahammed, 25, married but without children, lived in a camp on the outskirts of Beirut that was bombed three days ago. His house was destroyed. He speaks English and we can talk freely.

"Where will you go from here?" I ask, motioning to the city around.

"From here? We have nowhere to go."

"But the Israelis have dropped leaflets saying they are going to bomb Beirut and all the civilians should leave."

"We can't go anywhere else," he says in resignation. "There's no other place to go. If they bomb, that's just our fate."

An American in Lebanon feels indignation at first, then rage. Dennis went that route, too.

"In the past," he told me, "I would go to the States and give speeches about my view of the political situation. I don't care about that anymore. When you see suffering in such huge dimensions, you don't have time for that. You can be angry—my wife knows that I throw books against the wall when I read the dumb stuff that's written about the Middle East. And I shout when I hear lies on the radio. But now, I just want to be here to help as many people as possible."

He sent word to his friends in the United States:

"Don't talk to me about the political or military side of the tragedy. That's the problem of governments.

"Talk to me rather about the thousands of people wounded and dying, afraid and alone, sleepless and nervous, hungry and homeless, lost and orphaned, confused and abandoned. Talk to me about how we have been called by our Lord to speak Christ's message and presence to them. That's *my* problem."

And mine.

The blood of Ein-el-Hilweh and Kineye School of Tyre and Sidon of Sabra and Shatila cries out. Not for revenge. But for reconciliation worthy of such terrible sacrifice.

Christ, I am convinced, is on the side of healing.

I want to be where He is. Even if that *is* just a yard from hell.

7

A Place to Live *Belesi*

New Guinea

The village of Niksek at the headwaters of the Sepik River in Papua New Guinea may not yet be the settlement nearest to heaven, but it is a very long way from the hell its people lived in just a short time ago.

In case you should want to check out my statement for yourself, I'll give you directions. First, fly to Port Moresby, capital of the newly-independent Pacific nation. You can go via either Sydney or Manila, since it's roughly the same distance from each. Actually, the country of Papua New Guinea is one-half of the world's second largest island after Greenland. The western half, called Irian Jaya, belongs to Indonesia.

From Port Moresby, charter a small plane and head northwest. You'll fly over the Western Highlands and a central mountain range, with some of the highest peaks in the Pacific—nearly 15,000 feet. After about three hours you'll drop down into the government outpost of Ambunti, which sits on a slight elevation in the middle of limitless swamp forests.

You can take a boat from Ambunti to Niksek if you can

find someone willing to make the trip. That is unlikely, however, and not recommended because the trip would take the better part of two days and the river is treacherous.

Since it is impossible to walk from Ambunti—the jungle is literally trackless—your only other option would be to see if you could get the small two-passenger helicopter, operated by the Summer Institute of Linguistics, popularly known as the Wycliffe Bible Translators, to come from the mission's base and ferry you in.

Out of practical necessity that's how we did it; but I must confess my deep feelings of ambivalence at being set down in the midst of a Stone Age environment by a twentieth-century machine. It seemed, at the very least, we should have trekked or rowed the last few miles to soften the culture shock.

I've heard of places time forgot. This spot on the April River, one of the tributaries of the mighty Sepik, goes them one better. I had the feeling that time never found it.

It wasn't "found," in fact, until 1973 when a government patrol pushed its way past the known frontiers in a census-taking effort that preceded independence. That was the first time any outsider had laid eyes on the wild and rugged land except from the air. Even the mighty battles of World War II that raged over New Guinea had never touched this untamed jungle. It had been left to wild boar, crocodiles, the magnificent bird of paradise, and a primitive people who wore grass mini-skirts and sea shells on a G-string, grew taro and hunted wild boar, and lived by the law of *tambaran* and payback.

These were the Niksek and other tribal cousins. Although untouched by the outside world, they had through occasional contacts with other tribes learned about missionaries and had seen evidence of the change that comes to a society touched by these dedicated servants of Jesus Christ. They sent word out by the patrol that they would welcome such a person to come and live among them.

It was not until nearly three years later that word eventually got to Fritz Urschitz, a missionary with the Liebenzell Mission from Germany, who had already pioneered in two other areas. His mission agreed to lend him to the South Sea Evangelical Mission so that he could respond to the new challenge.

Fritz established a base at Ambunti and started building a house for his family. He was also planning his strategy, praying all the time for God to give him an opening up the river. The answer came dramatically when he met a man from the April River district who was in Ambunti as a witness in a court case. Nasam could speak Neo-Melanesian, or pidgin, the trade language of the country. When he discovered that Fritz was a missionary, he urged the 14-year veteran to open a work in his area.

So here was the invitation! But there was also the house to be built. Nasam agreed to stay and help with the construction if Fritz would accompany him upriver when the house was finished.

Deal!

The two men, accompanied by two national evangelists from another area, made the first boat trip in 1976. The patrol's message had been right. Weary of the superstitions and fears that bound them to the past, the Niksek people wanted to change. Through interpreters, the three outsiders spoke at length that first night about God, His creation and Jesus Christ. The people were so hungry for more spiritual knowledge that they kept the tired travelers up until 2:00 A.M., plying them with questions.

Says Fritz, "I trembled with excitement and could scarcely sleep the rest of the night!"

The people were so eager for more teaching that they

wanted their own resident missionary. And they wanted contact with the rest of the world. They desired both so badly, in fact, that they started carving an airstrip out of virgin jungle with nothing more than hand tools—bush knives and axes.

That was in 1977, and nearly two years later it was still only half-finished. Fritz had added a few spades and some files to their meager inventory of hand tools, as well as a small tractor, contributed by a church in Europe and brought upstream through great hazards on a government jet barge.

But the huge trees—up to a hundred feet tall and four to five feet in diameter—must still be felled by hand. And the massive stumps must be grubbed out and moved the same way.

Watching about two dozen men perform these nearly superhuman feats in the steaming heat of a tropical sun, I marveled at the motivation that had kept them going to clear that one-mile strip of jungle.

We talked about it that night after a pig feast and *sing-sing*—dancing by the warriors. The pig was a wild boar killed that morning and cooked on hot stones. Fritz had brought rice to mix with those native taro roots, which made it a banquet indeed for the Niksek whose usual diet consists almost solely of the starchy tuber grown in small clearings in the jungle.

Although I had eagerly anticipated sampling the wild boar, I yielded to the wiser judgment of a colleague who had been a missionary in the country for 20 years. He suggested that we stick to the canned salmon Fritz had thoughtfully brought along to spare both our molars and our digestive systems.

Reluctantly, I passed up the wild boar.

After the *sing-sing,* the group sent about 10 men over for *tok-tok*—Pidgin English for "talk-talk" or discussion.

We couldn't all fit into the little shack where we were spending the night, so they spilled out the doorway into the darkness.

The next two hours was for me a window into their world. We talked of many things, including the airstrip, but primarily of their past and future.

The past could be summed up in one pidgin phrase: "Me friat tumas," phonetically spoken as "Me fright too much" or roughly translated, "We were always filled with great fear." They spoke of the things that dominated and troubled them in the past—primarily the *sanguma*, the *tambaran*, poison and the rainworm.

The rainworm?

This small worm which lives in the ground was a god to them. If one was killed accidentally or harmed in any way, someone in the family would die. They know now this was a great superstition, and they've been liberated from this fear, but imagine the terror they felt each time they dug taro, fearing they might harm a god and thus a loved one!

The *sanguma* was the sorcerer. Because he controlled the powers of darkness and light, he exercised enormous power over the lives of the people.

The *tambaran* was the power of the enemy gods, and the enemy was everyone outside the immediate clan. And because everyone outside the immediate family is considered an enemy, poison—either from the enemy or from some outside spiritual source—was considered a constant threat. So families—perhaps 30 or 40 people—will huddle together in a huge "tall house" built in a tree some 30 feet off the ground to protect themselves against the enemy who lives over the hill or across the river.

The society had been one of fractured relationships. That is why few large villages exist where the gospel has not liberated the people from their fear of each other.

The entire culture was permeated with these primal

fears that affected everything, from the way they build houses to the way they hunted wild boars. A system of taboos—some food was forbidden to women, for example, and superstitions—a man who stayed in the same house with a menstruating woman would get asthma—was built up around these fears.

A man called John spoke first: "So many of the things we did were wrong and have not been helpful to us."

Jacob said he wanted to thank the missionary who brought this change to them. "Before, we didn't sit down well," he commented in the local idiom, "but now we sit down happy."

One of the men who speaks pidgin used the word *belesi*. The language is very picturesque. Pronounced *bell-easy,* the word could literally be translated, "a calm feeling in the stomach"; the stomach is the seat of the emotions in the Niksek culture. The English equivalent would be "our heart is at peace."

When I asked what are the advantages here in the village over life in the jungle, Nathan answered for them all: "Because God is here."

I was touched by these simple but eloquent descriptions of life on the banks of the April River.

To get an even deeper feeling of what the former life was like, I spent much of the next morning with a man named Abraham and his wife, Makana. The men's Bible names, I discovered, were not the work of the missionary. The people themselves had heard from other tribes of the practice of adopting a biblical name at the time of conversion and baptism since their infant names were often associated with animistic ceremonies. The village is now a veritable lexicon of Bible names!

Abraham, whose pre-Christian name was Sinae, told me about growing up. At the age of seven he began the five stages of initiation into manhood, which were not completed until he was 19. The initiation procedures were meant not only to prove his manhood to the tribe, but also to teach him to endure pain and to develop the qualities of a warrior. During these years he was also introduced to the gods and deities who would control his life.

The first stage for young Sinae was getting to know the *tumbunu,* the ways of his forefathers. Since the people have no recorded history, it must be handed down orally from generation to generation. For Sinae, this meant listening to the older men tell of great battles and brave warriors, of wild boar hunts and feuds with enemies.

The second stage was a continuation of the first until he was saturated with tribal lore.

When he was 14, Sinae was made to spend the night alone in the *huas tambaran,* the spirit house. In it were spirit fetishes, mementos of some of the battles he had heard about, the skulls as well as weapons of some of the great warriors, and the jawbones of scores of slain boars. The next morning he was taken out and made to run the "gauntlet of pain," in which he was slapped and lashed by the older men who, when he was a child, had been gentle with him. This taught him his new relationships in the adult world. After this third stage, he was no longer a boy, but he was also not yet a man.

The fourth step came when he was 19. Then he was taken back to the *huas tambaran,* this time to sit for two weeks with no food except sugarcane. The medicine men came and taught him tribal custom and law, especially the law of payback from which he has not yet been totally set free. It is basically the law of revenge—an eye for an eye and a tooth for a tooth. Only by practicing payback can a man retain his manhood.

During these two weeks he wove into his own hair some of the hair of his dead ancestors so that he might receive something of their *mana,* their life force.

At the end of this religious fasting period, Sinae had to go out and kill one of the enemy, thus demonstrating that the tribal gods were with him. He brought back a limb of the victim and took it into the spirit house where he ate the flesh and blood, thus taking into himself the warrior qualities of his victim.

Had he failed at any of these crucial test points during his initiation, the women would have taunted and ridiculed him, a fate so devastating to his pride that he would have been driven to suicide or to some spectacular feat to prove his manhood.

Stage five was the graduation ceremony, the public recognition of his rights as a man—the right to have land, own pigs, get a woman and have children. The climax was a giant *sing-sing* when his acceptance as a man was affirmed by the tribe.

That took place probably 30 years ago (we could only guess at his age), but it has shaped Sinae's life ever since. I asked him what his adult life had been like in the jungle.

"The old days were not good days," he began. "We walked in fear—fear of both man and the spirits who meant to do us harm. Even knowing the ways of our forefathers did not bring us peace. We would have a war, some would get killed, then we would make friends. But even after the friendship feast, we knew the enemy would be coming back to get us. And we looked for ways to get them. We did not know how to live together in the same forest."

In early 1978, Sinae heard about the new village on the April River where people were settling down *belesi*. When Fritz put up his simple building in 1977 it was the first hut around. Gradually, the people began to come. In less than two years, there were 21 huts and a population of about 180, including 30 members of one family living in a traditional "tall house," their own concession to the ancient life-style. New families were coming at the rate of about one a week. The chiefs had turned no one away.

The fame of the village spread as the number of families grew, and Sinae's heart hungered for what he heard was happening on the April River. So he started out for Niksek. Just on the other side of the river from the village, he was attacked by a wild boar and nearly killed. Bleeding heavily, he managed to climb a vine that was hanging from a branch; he stayed in the tree until the animal left.

A young boy heard his cries and he was taken across to Niksek by canoe. Thinking he would die, the people started their traditional wailing. Daniel, an evangelist who had returned to live in Niksek after his first trip with Fritz, quieted them and led them in prayer for the man. The only thing he could do was wash the gaping wounds with hot water.

Somehow, the injured man stayed alive until Fritz came a week later with penicillin. Sinae fully recovered. He and the people acknowledged that it was the true God who heard their prayers.

A year later, he and Makana were baptized in the April River along with 64 others, two of whom were Fritz's oldest sons.

Sinae became Abraham. I asked him what were his hopes for his children. He told me his two daughters will likely follow the traditional ways and marry as soon as they find the right men. As for his two sons, he said, "I do not want them to follow in the old ways of their forefathers. Those ways have proven to be wrong. I want them to have this new life. When I hear the 'book Bible' read, I know this is God talking. What God says is now the number one something in our lives."

Earlier that morning I had joined with other Christians in the village to hear God talk to us from the "book Bible." They come together for hymn singing and Bible study every morning at eight o'clock. If the weather is clear, they meet outside. If rain threatens, as it did that morning, they climb the 30-foot ladder to the "tall house." Its dimensions are about 20 by 40 feet, and I looked with some apprehension at the thin stilts supporting it, wondering if they might collapse under the weight of nearly a hundred people.

The stilts held. What the house may lack in architectural style it makes up in sturdiness, although I am told it rocks and sways precariously when sing-sings are held in it.

That morning Fritz spoke from Mark's Gospel on the two great commandments: "Thou shalt love the Lord thy God with all thy heart, and with all thy soul, and with all thy mind, and with all thy strength . . . and thou shalt love thy neighbor as thyself."

He emphasized the difference between their old life when they feared the bad spirits, and their new life centered around a God who is love. And he told them God commands them not to hate or fear others, but to love them. He spoke of the centuries-old law of payback and told them this is contrary to God's greater law. The words were especially appropriate, for there had been some recent experiences of injustices and wrongs done by those outside the village, and the new Christians had been debating whether or not they should retaliate.

Fritz sees the new attitudes gradually taking over and prays that none of the weaker believers will be tempted back into the old ways. When I discussed this with the men during our tok-tok, they told me, "We do not want to do payback killings. If other families do us wrong, we would rather be paid in shells or pigs. We are trying to learn the new way."

One of the songs we sang that morning was "Lord, I'm Coming Home." I thought it a remarkably fitting theme for these seminomadic people who have wandered the remote regions of New Guinea for centuries in search of a place to belong. Suspicions drove them farther from each other and fear sent them deeper into the jungle. No place was home for more than two years.

Now, there on the banks of the April River, isolated by swamp forests and the jungle vastness, a community of faith is being formed by the supernatural work of the Holy Spirit. A people who were not a people are finding new life together. That's something their forefathers, for countless generations, were never able to experience.

The Niksek people are at last beginning to find their way home where they can "sit down happy" and live *belesi*.

8

Long Road Home to Shaba

Zaire

The old man had arrived in Kasaji the previous day, the same day I came to Kolwezi. He looked in pretty bad shape, so I moved over to talk to him. Below his ragged shorts, his legs were badly swollen and his black skin had that shiny, unhealthy look.

I wondered how old he was. He said he didn't know. I asked him, "How many people came back with you?"

"Many." (To illiterate people, any numbers over the few needed to count children or chickens become "many.")

Actually, I found out that some 200 returning refugees had made it back to Kasaji the day before. Another 600 had crossed the border at Dilolo. The trickle had become a stream.

It had taken him one month to walk from Angola. His swollen legs had made each step an agonizing experience. His infected left hand was tied up in a small, dirty sling and pain was etched into the lines of his face.

Why did you come back?

He acted as if the question were foolish, which it probably was. His answer was given matter-of-factly and with a touch of finality in his voice: "We must return to our homes."

The long road had finally brought him back home. Home to Shaba.

Along with an estimated 250,000 others, he had fled his home province in Zaire, formerly known as the Belgian Congo, 16 months before when *les tigres*—the tigers—came over the border from Angola in one more attempt to wrest the copper-rich province, formerly Katanga, away from Zaire. The battle has gone on with varying degrees of intensity since Zaire gained its independence from Belgium in 1960.

As long as there was a Portuguese presence in Angola, which borders the Zairian province on the south, the Katangese rebels were pretty much kept in check. But with the establishment of a Marxist regime in Luanda in 1976, the Shaba conflict heated up.

First, there was the invasion of 1977, called "Shaba I" or the "Eighty-Day War." A number of towns in the south-western part of the province were occupied for several weeks. A Methodist missionary doctor was murdered after being put through a show trial. But apart from that single incident involving a foreigner, it was mostly the blacks who suffered. That didn't make many headlines in Western newspapers.

Then in 1978 came Shaba II. This invasion had as its main target the important mining center of Kolwezi, with a population of 100,000. This time the rebels massacred 131 whites and Shaba was catapulted to the front of international news. Both France and Belgium launched military operations to airlift the remaining 2,250 European technicians and their families to safety and free the city from its six-day occupation. The Americans gave logistical support to the operation.

Most of the massacred Europeans were shot in cold blood. It was a violent and unmistakable message to any foreigners who would come to help the national government operate the copper mines. The brutality shocked the world.

But the part of the story that got left out of the reporting was the greater suffering of the Africans themselves. In the same military operation, the African death toll was 589, including a Methodist pastor who was shot in his home. Between the terrorist activities of the rebels and the plundering of the Zairian army, most of the local villages had been stripped of virtually everything and left to face a bleak and uncertain future.

As with most of the conflicts I have seen all over the world, the little people are the ones who get shot up, burned out and driven away. They cannot fight back, protest or escape.

They can only suffer. And most of them don't even know the reasons why. The old man I was talking to in Kasaji had only the vaguest idea of what the fighting was all about. When I asked him why he ran away, his simple answer was: "I was afraid."

Fear still ruled the countryside. The rebels were gone, but because of tribal enmities that date back many generations and more recent political realities, the people are as afraid of the army as they are of the rebels.

Now another enemy had arrived—invisible, deadly and even more relentless than the others. Hunger. That is why I was in Shaba. To explore a relief program in cooperation with *Eglise du Christ au Zaire,* the Church of Christ in Zaire, a united church.

Until our survey team flew in, the only outsiders to visit Kolwezi after the massacre were Zairian military personnel. Getting permission to go was in itself a major hurdle, achieved only after intervention by Bishop Bokeleale, president of the *Eglise du Christ au Zaire.*

But an even greater obstacle was finding someone to take us there. Anybody who flew into Shaba risked losing a plane either by having the rebels shoot it down or the army confiscate it on the ground. When we revealed our destination there were no planes in Kinshasha available for charter. Except one.

The plane was an ancient DC-3 that had seen service with the Argentine Air Force. When it was retired, it had found its way to Africa and wound up in the hands of an American soldier of fortune. Used for whatever licit or illicit traffic was available, the owner agreed to use his antique craft to fly us to Shaba under one condition: he had to be paid in dollars rather than local currency.

That would make it possible for him to buy a rebuilt engine the plane badly needed. An agreement was struck and we took off the next morning on one good engine, one bad engine and a lot of prayer.

We had a passenger load of 12 people plus 2,200 pounds of milk powder and emergency food as well as six drums of fuel for the return flight.

It was too much for an aircraft with a limp. "We'd better take off some of the food," the pilot said, "or else we're not going to make it."

With the load lightened, he was more optimistic, but not without a couple of anxiety-producing caveats: "If we can clear the end of the runway and if we can climb a few feet, we'll make it."

As the plane lumbered from Kinshasa to Kolwezi, a five-and-a-half hour experience, I became aware of the immensity of the country. Zaire covers about the same amount of territory as the entire United States east of the Mississippi River.

Even as we approached the airport at Kolwezi, I could see something of what had taken place during the invasion.

Burned-out skeletons of planes, including two that belonged to the Methodist mission, lay scattered around the parking area. The tower had been shot up methodically. In an effort to paralyze the city and prevent immediate assistance, the rebels had targeted their objectives well.

We buzzed the city a couple of times to announce our presence and, sure enough, when we landed there was a big welcoming party. On hand were Bishop Ngoy, head of the Methodist Church in Shaba; Carroll French, a Methodist agriculturist who had just returned the day before with his wife and two children; Terry Smith, a British Brethren missionary; and Ward Williams, another Methodist missionary who served as administrator for the bishop. The bishop's pilot, Stan Ridgeway, was there also with a small plane from Lubumbashi, the provincial capital.

Among other logistical problems to be solved once we were on the ground was the problem of where to find beds and food for so many visitors in a ghost town. We finally wound up in a house that had been abandoned by a European family but was still pretty much intact.

In the villages near Kolwezi we were able to see one side of the problem. The people here had lived in relative security until the last round of fighting. When the invasion came by *les tigres,* followed by the army counterattack, they fled to the bush. Only after three months did they feel safe enough to start returning to their homes.

I talked with the chief of Tshabula, a village of 400 inhabitants six miles from Kolwezi. They all left when the fighting started, he said, and only 140 have returned. The morning we were there, just a few were around. The rest had gone to search for food, and a few who had salvaged their hoes were working in gardens near the little stream close by the village.

But the moment we arrived, I felt something strange

about Tshabula. The mood was subdued, almost eerie.
The thing gnawed at me, but I couldn't identify it. What
was it?

Then suddenly it hit me. There were no children! Not
a single one. It was such an unusual experience that I
rushed to one of the missionaries and asked, "Where are
the children?"

I've been in hundreds of villages all over the world and
never have I failed to be surrounded by scores and sometimes hundreds of children. Not only do they add to the
noise level, but their presence puts a dynamism in village
life. Without them, Tshabula seemed lifeless.

The mystery was soon solved.

"The war has made the children afraid," the chief told
us. "They don't want to be away from their parents so
they go with them everywhere."

Sure enough, we saw them later—even boys up to 12
years old—staying very close to their mothers, whether
they were in the gardens or scrounging for food. They
were like frightened fawns.

I thought, "What terrible sins are inflicted upon the
innocence and joy of childhood by mankind's monstrous
wickedness."

The situation in Tshabula was bad. Almost as bad as
anything I've seen. Most of the mud shacks had been
looted and burned. Not more than half-a-dozen cooking
pots were left in the whole village. It was the same with
hoes.

But the food situation was the worst problem. Most
families normally would have some grain stored in the tops
of their shacks for use in hard times. This, too, had been
taken. The final indignity and tragedy was that the manioc
fields had been pulled up and destroyed.

Manioc, a starchy tuber, is the diet staple. Destroying
a field shows malicious intent to destroy a people, because

it takes three years to grow a new crop.

"In the past," the chief said, "when a thief would come into our houses to steal, we would find the person and cut off his hands. But what can we do? The people who do these things have guns and we are helpless."

It was obvious that his reference to "the people" meant both sides.

He showed me the consequence of powerlessness. In one of the few remaining pots was a couple of handfuls of leaves. That would be his meal today. It was also what he had eaten yesterday. The same is true for most of the people. Some days they are able to buy a little manioc or corn meal, but mostly now they live on the leaves of bushes and vines.

Besides being poor in nutrition and without taste, the chief told me, the leaves caused people to have stomach problems.

An hour's flight away, in Kasaji, things are not much different. This is where the people have been away from their villages for nearly 18 months. When they come back from Angola, as had the old man I talked to, they also find their homes looted and burned. The animals are gone. The fields are grown over. And life must be started all over again at square one.

But in spite of it all, they are glad to be home in Shaba. In Angola, they told me, life was even more bitter. They lived in the bush and no one came to help them. They ate leaves there, too, and many died from starvation.

"Hunger is the worst thing," they said. "It bites at the stomach."

Nearly every family I talked to had buried at least one member in Angola. Muzanga Koji watched his wife die, knowing there was nothing he could do for her. Standing next to him was 24-year-old Mujinga Tshisola who had given birth to her first child in the bush. Her eyes filled with tears as she spoke her quiet faith: "I know God looked after us over there."

Many gave the same testimony and I saw great faith in spite of the great suffering. In deep trial, they had never doubted God. Seventy percent of the people of Shaba profess Christianity, 40 percent Catholic and 30 percent Protestant.

They still believe God will help them now that they are back home, but they don't know how. The most urgent need, after each day's food, is hoes for cultivation.

I still think about the old man with the swollen legs. I asked him what he needed most. That created a lot of discussion from the crowd around us. They sounded like the audience at a television game show, advising the contestant how to choose. Most of them told him to ask for clothes. Although I couldn't quite tell because of all the commotion, I think his wife also was encouraging him to opt for clothes.

I must confess there was a great deal of logic in their choice. His brown shorts were in tatters. They were the same ones he had worn the day he left Kasaji for refuge in Angola. He had no shirt. The ragged shorts were the only piece of clothing he owned.

He listened until the chatter quieted. Then he looked at me and said, "Give me a hoe!"

And he would not be dissuaded.

I marked a hoe for him on the first planeload of supplies flown in from Kenya. But I never had a chance to go back and find out if he received it. I took the staff's word for it that the relief program had been successful.

The decision not to go back to Kolwezi didn't even require a second thought. I would like to have seen the people again, but I had no desire to spend any time in the local jail. And most likely, that's what would have happened.

When I heard the news a month later, I tried to be philosophical about the fact that my name was on the arrest list in Shaba Province. Not that I had expected to win any popularity contests with the army when I told a colonel—who kept terrorizing the villagers by waving his automatic weapon in their faces—to butt out, only I used stronger words.

Nonetheless, I did think the order to arrest me if I set foot back in the province was something of an overreaction. But since discretion is said to be the better part of valor, I decided to be discreet and not go back.

The first time had been exciting. I wasn't sure I could handle the boredom of a jail cell.

9

One Drought from Death

Ethiopia

Landing this bucket of bolts would be the trickiest part of the whole trip, I thought apprehensively as I looked out the window.

Reason: There was no airstrip below.

The flight from Addis Ababa had taken something over three hours, allowing for the fuel stop at Arba Minch. Now we were coming in low over an unmarked piece of desert in Ethiopia's southwest corner.

But our 40-year-old DC-3 touched down on the sun-baked earth as gently as if it had been the main runway on an international airport. The pilot of the plane, one of two ancient aircraft belonging to the government's Relief and Rehabilitation Commission (RRC), knew his business.

We taxied toward a line of trees along a dried-up river-bed where from the air we had seen hundreds of *mutuls,* the domeshaped huts of sticks and grass typical of nomadic peoples in the Horn of Africa. The plane stopped, the engines were throttled to silence, the door was opened, a ladder was clamped into place—and I swung down into one of the most challenging experiences of my life.

More than 2,000 Bume (pronounced Boo-may) tribes-people, mostly women and children, had gathered in the shade of a huge acacia tree; more were streaming to the tree from their huts which were grouped together behind a protecting thorn barricade.

While they gathered, we walked to what remained of the river, hearing at every step stories of incredible suffering that had befallen the Bume during the drought. Mothers, their breasts dry and sagging, are feeding their children roots when they can find them, and leaves of a tree they get from the mountain which is a half-day's walk away. It takes 8 to 10 hours to cook the bitter leaves to edibility; they contain little nourishment and cause diarrhea.

We are in the province of Gamo-Gofa, at the point where Ethiopia, Kenya and Sudan meet. Of the nine provinces in trouble, Gamo-Gofa is one of the worst hit. The numbers are staggering—400,000 people in this province alone face disaster; 5 million in the whole country.

Since 1973, the Bume have lived only one drought away from death. Now the rains have failed again. *Newsweek* calls it East Africa's "worst drought in 15 years."

As we come to a dry riverbed, I ask, "What do they do for water?" Then I see the deep pits that have been dug in the river bottom. The only tools for digging are the omnipresent gourds, which are also used to collect food and keep the blistering sun's rays off the head.

We walk to the edge of one pit. Thirty feet down are a couple of inches of muddy water. A week ago, for the first time in two years, a brief shower provided a short-lived respite. But the ground is parched again—only this scant residue remains. The trees along the empty river will soon again turn brown and sere.

The only reliable source of water is the Kibish River

into which this branch drains five miles away. Families make the 10-mile round trip when the water holes here dry up.

Like now.

While we watch, a small boy, wearing nothing but a brave smile, scrambles down into the pit and with his hands scoops up a mouthful of dirty water.

When we return to the acacia tree, more people have assembled. I begin to get a clue as to their expectations when the children set up a chant. I ask if they are saying "Good morning." Somebody tells me they are asking for food.

Two officials from the RRC, Ato Tamaru and Ato Bekele ("Ato" is Amharic for "Mr.") tell me, "For the last four years these people have been struggling. They have lost their cattle, their goats, their sheep. Now people are dying because they depend on their animals for food. The government is trying to help, but because of the distance and the needs in so many other provinces, keeping people alive here is very difficult."

The people ask me to say something. I tell them we are committed to feed hungry people as an act of Christian love. I tell them they are our brothers and sisters and that I will inform the world about their needs.

One of the chiefs then speaks to me. His words have to be translated in reverse—from Bume to Amharic to English. He said simply: "When there is no rain, there are no cattle. When there are no cattle, there is no food. When there is no food, there will be no people. You are looking at a dying people who will be gone in a few weeks if we do not get food today."

"Please don't wait until next week," he added, "because we cannot last that long."

I was still feeling the weight of his words and wondering what we could do about the situation when I had another eventful encounter. This one was with a woman named Amila, perhaps in her early forties. Wearing a cattle hide draped over one shoulder, another skin tied around her waist, bracelets on ankles and wrists, two small children in tow, she pushes her way through the crowds and stands facing me.

She carries an empty gourd bowl. As she begins speaking accusingly, someone translates. I will never forget what she says: "When we saw the plane coming this morning, we thought you were bringing food. We walked with empty stomachs to this relief center, and we didn't get anything. We saw only you."

I feel there is no need for me to try to explain there was no way we could have brought food with us, especially not for 16,000 people who live—perhaps "exist" is a better word—in just this one area of Gamo-Gofa. We had come to survey now and planned to send food later. The government had been most cooperative in making this plane available to us.

I didn't say any of that. Hungry people can't eat explanations.

Amila has more to say, and as she says it, she wags her finger inches from my face: "You have told us a lot. You have promised us a lot. I don't want you to forget what you have told us. I want you to prove it in action. Please, please do not forget us."

I tell this earnest woman: "My heart will not allow me to forget. I promise in the name of God that as quickly as we can get a plane here with food, you and your children will eat."

I didn't know how we would do it, only that it had to be done. Empty hands are no answer to empty stomachs.

Amila started to dance slowly and to sing. The other women with children joined her and someone told me what they were singing: "Today our father has come. We thought we would die. We thought our children would die. But we are going to eat. Our children are going to live, because today our father has come."

It was a song they made up as they went along. Talk about having it laid on you! By faith, I had promised food in the name of God. The people believed me, but I knew it was up to God to protect His name. I had no human way to do it.

We talked together—the RRC officials, my colleagues and I. If we would buy the food and pay the cost of the plane, the RRC officials agreed to distribute food the next day. Without even asking how much it would cost, I agreed. Even though there was no budget for this extra program there was no question but that we had to meet the crisis.

The next morning we flew back to the desert from Arba Minch, the provincial capital, a town of 7,600, where lions sometimes wander into town from the surrounding open spaces, and people talk about the bush cobra that rises vertically and remains still until prey comes within reach.

Amila was waiting, along with scores of other families. When she saw me, she raised her hand slowly and started to shuffle toward me. As I moved to meet her, I raised my own hand and we joined them in a touching greeting.

She points to her stomach as she talks to me in Bume. I don't understand the words, but I don't need to. I respond, "Yes, today you and your children eat."

After each family registers, an allotment is made: 15 kilograms of maize for each adult, 7.5 kilos for each child. In addition, 3 kilos of fortified food for each nursing mother and malnourished child, plus 1.5 kilos of butter oil for each family.

As the distribution continues, children pick up every stray kernel of corn, some immediately popping them into their mouths, some hoarding the treasure in small tin cans. An old grandmother is on her knees in the dust where a few handfuls have fallen, scooping them together into her skin cape and then carefully separating them from the dirt, kernel by kernel.

Senior deputy administrator of Gomo-Gofa, Gebre Kidan Amare, tells me that although water is the basic need here, drilling has not proven very successful. He believes it would be possible to pipe water from the Kibish River to a point where the people might be resettled. They cannot live by the river itself because of the tsetse flies.

Then he says, "Nomads do not move for the sake of moving. That is a misconception. They move simply to reach water. The people need food, clothing, medicines and specialized feeding for the children. There are immediate needs, but water is the big need. With water, the people can become self-sufficient."

I promise that we will survey for a possible resettlement program.

We visit Amila's hut before we leave. She shows us how she grinds roots on a flat stone, using another stone as a pestle. She puts her cowhide cape underneath to catch any morsel that falls. She has 10 children, but two are dead. It has been two years since her cattle perished. Her husband died seven years ago, but now she has another husband and that explains why she has young children.

Five people live in Amila's tiny *mutul*. The smallest children stay inside at night; the others sleep outside.

She says, "When we had herds, we had milk, and when it rained, we could plant sorghum. Since the rains stopped we have been suffering all the time."

I tell her it was her strong speech yesterday that caused the food to be provided today. She thanks us for the food today, but says she worries about the future.

"What will we do when this is gone?" Amila asks, pointing to her sack of grain.

"We will remember you," I promise Amila again, and stand up to leave. "I will not let the world forget."

She continues to sit, holding the littlest child on her lap. "Go in peace," she says.

It is a poignant farewell.

But as we return to the plane, I wonder how one *can* go in peace from this sad little corner of Ethiopia.

10

"You Came Back"

Ethiopia

She's coming," someone yelled.

I had been dozing in the shade of an acacia tree on the bank of the Kibbish River in southwestern Ethiopia, resting from the oppressive heat.

Roused by the cry, I climbed the embankment separating once-fertile fields from the bone-dry river. At the top of the short ridge, I could see a puff of dust in the distance. Someone was running toward me across the barren field. A woman.

I recognized her and hoped she would remember me. I hoped she would be pleased that I had gone home and told millions of my people about the plight of her people, the Bume.

My listeners responded in an unprecedented manner and much of the credit goes to one courageous woman—Amila.

You remember Amila.

She was the woman who came to me during my first visit to this remote corner of the world and demanded that I do more than just talk about starving people. I had come to this home of the nomads—right at the point where Ethiopia, Sudan and Kenya share a common border—to survey the devastating effects of a three-year drought.

The land was parched. The cattle were dead, their carcasses rotting in the sun. With the loss of cattle and subsistence crops, the people were starving. All they had to eat were bitter leaves and dry roots scavenged from hillsides far beyond the horizon. In a land where the average temperature often soars above 90 degrees, scavenging for food in distant places, with no water to quench thirst, can be deadly in itself.

I had seen the need and was ready to return home to share it with others. Then out of the crowd came Amila. She had a different idea about what my plan should be. And her voice sounded to me like the voice of God.

"When we saw the plane coming this morning, we thought you were bringing food," she said accusingly, waving a bony finger close to my face. "We walked with empty stomach to this relief center and we didn't get anything. We saw only you."

Her eyes pierced my soul with conviction. I knew I couldn't leave this hungry, disappointed woman and 16,000 more villagers with vague promises about a relief program someday. So I told her we'd have food there the quickest way possible, and I promised it in the name of God. I didn't know what we would do; I knew only that we had to do something.

Through an arrangement with the Ethiopian Relief and Rehabilitation Commission (RRC), we fulfilled that commitment. I returned to Bume the very next day with food!

Amila had called me her father after that, for the father in Bume society is the person who provides food for his family. Through an act of Christian kindness, done on behalf of thousands of caring people, I had suddenly become father to a tribe of African nomads! Maybe that helps you understand why I had to come back to Ethiopia—to see Amila and my "family."

As I rested on the river bank, waiting for Amila, I flashed back on all the good news I had to tell her. About the funds we had raised. About nurses. Supplemental feedings. Resettlement villages. About cotton cloth and blankets. And about the airplane we had bought.

Just this morning, as I arrived at the airport in Addis Ababa, the Ethiopian capital, the new plane's pilot, Dave Schlener, met me. As we talked, he told me the Twin Otter has a short takeoff and landing capability—perfectly suited to rough runways and difficult weather. The plane can carry 22 passengers or a payload of 2.2 metric tons.

"We are now making six runs a day between our base camp at Mizan Tiveri and the village of Mardur where the Srumah people live," Dave told me excitedly. "We are trying hard, sir, to become more efficient so we can make seven runs a day."

We flew from Addis to the crew's base at Mizan, where we picked up several nurses. Then it was on to Mardur. The medical team is very important to the relief program because malnutrition leaves in its wake a series of devastating diseases. So as soon as we had put together a plan to rush food to the people of Ethiopia, we also started recruiting medical personnel.

Joan Smedley is an Australian, formerly with the Church Missionary Society, who worked among the aborigines in her own country for 20 years. I talked with her at Mardur as she tenderly cared for an emaciated infant.

"When you were here several months ago, there were 11,000 people waiting for food at this camp," she reminded me. "Now there are only 1,000 and they are seriously ill. Because of the quick response, the others are receiving food rations that make it possible for them to go back to their homes in the bush between distributions."

I asked Joan about conditions among those people who remained at the camp.

"Many are still sick, like this baby. He may not live. His mother's milk is all dried up. She, too, is in poor health, probably related to all those months without food."

I asked Joan about other diseases prevalent at Mardur. "Many related to malnutrition," she told me, "such as worms, diarrhea, even some tuberculosis. A decent diet would go a long way toward solving most of these problems. Unfortunately, it has been a long time since these people ate the kind of meal you and I take for granted."

Joan said that here at Mardur she had learned firsthand just how precious water is. "To clean wounds and mix formulas and medicine, we need clean water," she related, "but there just isn't any. We either have to bring water on the airplane each day or use the local supply from a stagnant pool about half-a-mile away. When the pool isn't dry, the water is muddy and contaminated so we have to use purification tablets in it."

Joan's colleague, Grace Ampah from Ghana, also talked about the challenges of treating patients here. "It is difficult to diagnose a person's problems given the language barrier," she noted. "We sometimes need a person to translate from English to Amharic, the national Ethiopian language. They, in turn, tell someone who speaks Amharic and Srumanya, the local language. Then we have to go through the process again in reverse, all for a simple explanation like, 'I have a headache.' Thank God for His grace that supplies us with patience."

Scores of children were walking around with big yellow bowls. Every child with such a bowl was entitled to three—sometimes four—meals a day from the supplemental feeding program. The effort is run by Esther Manieson, another nurse from Ghana.

As I wandered through the camp, Esther was instructing several naked children how to properly stir the mixture of grain and powdered milk that was cooking in a huge black pot over an open fire.

Waiting patiently in line were many children, probably as many as one-third of the 600 children in camp. When the gruel was completed, they would get a portion of that life-sustaining mixture.

"The children and mothers are so thankful we have arrived with this special feeding program," Esther told me. "You know, the other day I heard one child laugh. A deep belly laugh. Lord, that was a beautiful moment for me. Just to hear a child laugh!"

I understood.

The first time I visited Mardur, there was nothing but silence. The silence was made even more eerie by the fact that there were 11,000 people here, waiting for food distribution targeted for only a few hundred people. Most knew they had not registered in time to receive what little food was available, but there was no place else to go. So most of them sat silently outside the compound, silently awaiting the slow, torturous death of starvation.

I will never forget the frustration and anger I felt at being present where one human being was dying each hour simply because he or she had nothing to eat.

But this day, just a few months later, I found Mardur to be a different place. I had noticed it the moment I climbed out of the Twin Otter. Patches of green gave evidence that some rain had fallen, although not enough to break the drought. A few patches of corn had stalks that were five feet tall. The children walked more energetically; one was even running. It was obvious that our aid had made a profound difference in the once morgue-like atmosphere of Mardur.

On my previous visit, I had had an encounter very

much like the one with Amila down at Bume. This one had come from a dignified elder of the people. He hobbled out to the middle of the runway to say good-bye to me.

"Don't forget us," he implored.

I assured him I would not forget. And I drew him a picture in the dirt of a cross over a circle.

"When you see a plane returning with this symbol, you will know that I have kept my promise," I told him.

This day, some four months later, I was hoping I would still find the old gentleman alive.

I had already asked about two other people. One was a young mother with sad eyes who was suckling a dying child. The child had died even before we had left Mardur that first day. I was told that the mother, too, had died just a month later, leaving three orphaned children who had been taken to the resettlement village.

Then I asked about an old woman—65 pounds of skin and bones—who had collapsed at my feet. I had helped carry her to the shade of a nearby hut. "She, too, is dead," the camp leader told me.

So when I asked about old Dokuba Walazog, I expected to hear that he also had been buried in a simple hole in the ground in the midst of some small trees about a mile from the camp, like all the others.

When someone said they would go get him, I felt excitement begin to rise inside me. Of the three people, he was the one I least expected to see alive.

A few moments later he came, walking slowly with the aid of a stick, but still standing upright and proud. As before, he wouldn't let the younger men help him. Seeing me, he smiled ever so slightly and said gently, "You came back."

His simple words flooded my heart. How I thanked God he was still alive so I could share with him what God was doing to help the Srumah people.

"Yes, I've come," I told him. "Remember I told you when the plane came with the symbol that it would be from Christian brothers and sisters who cared, and it would mean that I had kept my promise because they made it possible."

"I remember," he said. "I even have this blanket from your airplane."

The gray blanket with red stripes was draped over his thin body. Dokuba then told me he was living in a little shelter by himself. Several family members, including three wives, were living just outside the camp. When the ration of five kilograms (11 pounds) of food per person per month was passed out—usually corn, powdered milk and *fafa*, a high protein grain mixture—he and his family received their ration together.

As we sat on a bench near his hut, I examined Dokuba's leg. It had been badly swollen four months before. Now the swelling was gone. Although badly scarred, it looked like it would heal.

My son, Eric, a photographer, took a few pictures with a Polaroid camera of Dokuba and me. When Eric gave Dokuba the exposed pictures, he watched in amazement as his image began slowly appearing on the once-blank paper.

A few friends gathered around, hoping to catch a peek at what was happening. Proudly Dokuba lifted the photo for all to see. One friend who wanted to touch it was quickly rebuffed. Dokuba didn't want anyone's hands on his treasured possession.

I walked away from Dokuba thinking about some of the younger people and wondered what their future might be. Beyond relief, what could be done to help the Srumah in the long term?

The Ethiopian government, thankfully, has embarked on an experimental program that may answer some of my concerns. They have transferred 500 Srumah to Mizan Tiferi for agricultural training. When we had stopped there to pick up the nurses, I had visited the center, accompanied by Bekele Asfew of the RRC. We were briefed by a camp leader who told us the people were learning to grow carrots, cabbage and different leafy vegetables. Normally the Srumah grow crops suited to their nomadic life-style—maize, millet and some sorghum.

The camp leader told us that at first the Srumah were resistant to any changes in their centuries-old life-style. "Once they tasted some of the vegetables they had grown, however, they changed their minds," he said.

Mr. Bekele and I talked with a 25-year-old Srumah man who had adopted the Amharic name, Bekele, also. His parents, four brothers and three sisters still lived near the camp at Mardur. He told me their cattle had died more than a year ago and they had barely survived, eating rations supplied by the RRC.

He had been at the agricultural camp six months. "I'm happy to be here," he said, "but I do miss my family."

Standing six feet tall without shoes, this strong, handsome man told me that when he arrived in camp, he was skin and bones. "I was very hungry," he said simply.

As Mr. Bekele and I moved on, the sounds of children reciting words from a blackboard drifted through the center of camp. Children and women are learning at school in the morning while the men are working in the fields. In the afternoon, the men take classes in reading and writing, as well as agricultural techniques.

I asked the government official what would happen to these people when they left here.

"We hope they will go to resettlement areas in Kaffa province," he said.

"Will the government supply the land?"

"Yes, that is our plan. Some of the people say they

would like to grow coffee, for which Kaffa province is famous, as a cash crop. Others want to continue being herdsmen. So we will put them into different projects and let them do what they want."

I was impressed by the vitality of the Srumah young people, and touched by their simplicity. While at Mardur, I sat down in the shade of one of the huts to rest briefly and was immediately surrounded by 8 or 10 youths. With no interpreter present, I couldn't converse with them so they talked among themselves. They stroked the hair on my arm, obviously intrigued by it since the Srumah have almost no body hair.

One of the camp leaders walked up and listened to their conversation.

"Do you know what they are saying?" he asked me.

I assured him I didn't.

Here's what he told me: "One of them said to the others, 'This man is our father.' When they inquired how could this be so, he asked them, 'What does your father do for you?' 'Why, he gives us food and shelter and takes care of us,' they replied. 'Since that is what this man does for us, then he is truly our father,'" the first one responded with what he was sure was irrefutable logic.

It was a tender moment for me as we came to the end of my return visit to Mardur.

My anticipation at meeting Amila was mounting. As soon as the pilot had shut off the engines, I had jumped onto the hard desert floor and began walking toward the Bume village.

Immediately I inquired of the village chief about Amila. She was in Kenya, I was told, on the other side of the Kibbish River, planting sorghum. Since it was quite hot, we decided to wait at a shady spot on the river bank while some boys ran to get her.

I was resting and reflecting at that spot when the shout

came that Amila was coming. She was on her way back.

Now, as the puff of dust became larger, I could see that
she was waving a green branch. It stood out beautifully
against the otherwise brown countryside. She was still
running. She had run all the way from her field, in stifling
heat, just to greet me. I was deeply moved.

We came together in a customary Bume greeting of
clasped hands. Although winded, she said over and over,
almost in a whimper, "Abba, Abba, Abba." Like the Srumah young people, this precious woman still considered
me her father.

A few moments later, after a drink of water from one
of my bottles, we sat in the shade and talked.

"I'm very glad to see you," I said. "How have you
been?"

"The children are sick," she said.

"I'm sorry. What were you planting in Kenya?"

"Sorghum. Far away there is some water."

"I have not forgotten our time six months ago," I
replied.

"I will never forget you either," she said.

"Many, many people all over the world heard your plea
for food and clothing for your children. Because of your
courage to confront me that day, thousands of people are
being helped all over Ethiopia."

She nodded and smiled. As we continued talking, Amila's eyes never left mine. Someone brought a blanket and a
bolt of cloth for her from the distribution center. I
explained this was a gift from people who love God and
love her.

I think she understood.

I wish I could tell you that our whole conversation was
a big happy reunion. But that would be naive, for there is
still heartbreaking need throughout Ethiopia. And an even

greater outpouring of love is required to meet those needs. Amila reminded me of this.

"Our water is muddy. Many children are still sick and hungry, like mine," she said. "We have skin sores because there is no animal fat to oil our leather clothing. Nor is there any oil for our hair. And there is still little food here at Bume. Some in my village will eat today; some won't."

"We will continue to help," I replied.

"We want to see our children grow up with fathers and families all together. I am very happy you have come to see us again," Amila said. Clasping hands again, we said good-bye.

As our plane circled Bume and Dave dipped the wings in salute, I saw Amila still waving. I thought about our first parting when she had told me, "Go in peace." That time I had left Bume full of uneasiness at the hopelessness and hunger I had seen.

This time I felt better. Life has been revived. Hope rekindled. Laughter restored. It felt glorious to be a part of that.

Having returned and seen it, I could now go in peace.

11

One More Gentle Miracle

Cambodia

His name was Chap (pronounced *chop*), but the relief worker didn't find that out at first.

In fact, at first he couldn't find out anything about the wild, dirty and ragged child who would hang around the small, open food stall on one of Phnom Penh's side streets. When he tried to approach the boy, Chap would run away.

The woman who ran the stall couldn't help. She told the relief worker that no one bothered with the boy except the other children who laughed at him. Twelve-year-old boys wandering alone in Cambodia's capital city are not a rare sight. The country has thousands of orphans, one of the awful legacies left by the genocidal Pol Pot.

But one day the foreign relief official got close enough to Chap to see that he was hiding a plastic bag under his ragged shirt and that in the bag were the boy's intestines.

He determined to bring the tragic case to the newly-opened pediatric hospital for which I had raised the funds, but he could never get close enough to Chap to talk to him and there were times when the boy would disappear for days. He was like a wild animal, hiding out in the deserted parks and abandoned buildings.

The woman at the food stall, one of the few Christian

believers left in Phnom Penh, had compassion for the boy and agreed to help the relief worker catch him. They succeeded, and that's how I happened to see Chap.

When Dr. Josianne André examined Chap, she discovered that he had been operated on sometime before and the incision had not healed. His intestines had spilled out through the hole.

But the boy would not talk—indeed, they believed he could not talk—in order to tell them what had happened to him. They can only surmise that the awful experiences of his young life, probably including seeing his parents killed by Khmer Rouge soldiers and his subsequent abandonment, had completely traumatized him and caused him to retreat emotionally and psychologically to the only safe place he knew—inside himself.

He had lost the ability to speak and to relate to other human beings.

Chap required major surgery, and since the medical facility was still without a surgeon, Dr. André took him to another hospital in the city where an East German surgical team agreed to operate.

While Chap waited for the operation, the Christian medical team visited him every day, but most often he was not in his bed. One day they found him hiding in the huge expanse of woods that surrounded the hospital. Confinement had been too much for his animal instincts.

But he recognized his new friends and was happy to see them. It seemed that he had taken his first step back toward being a human again. They gave him a new shirt to hide his plastic bag and took him back to await the urgently-needed operation.

The surgery was successful and after three days he was taken to the pediatric hospital for postoperative care and recovery from pneumonia. But having become used to the other hospital, Chap was not pleased to be transferred. He regressed into his wild ways.

Gradually, under the loving care of the staff, he ran away less often. But he still couldn't communicate. The doctors and nurses tried everything to break into his life. It happened one day when Nurse Michele Jeanrichard was coaxing him to count in French. He started to say the numbers after her and was so pleased with himself that he smiled for the first time.

Another breakthrough occurred when another nurse took Chap's picture. He loved that—and smiled all day.

Then when Dr. Marvin Raley went to visit his family in Singapore, he brought back from his son's toy box a wooden train. At first Chap didn't want to look at it, but after a while he reached out and touched it with the tip of his toe. Before long, he was pulling it up and down the hospital corridors.

Each small venture into the world outside that was met with acceptance seemed to encourage him to attempt another one. Soon the staff saw him bending over a crib where a small baby lay. He watched for a few minutes, then reached down gently and kissed the sleeping infant.

Some of the staff cried.

Chap still doesn't talk, but he smiles a lot now. However, even the shelter, food and love at the hospital haven't yet subdued his wanderlust. The day before I arrived, a member of the staff found him wandering around the grounds of the Royal Palace in his hospital pajamas. He had walked four miles to get there! Later in the day, he walked back by himself.

Every day gentle miracles like Chap are taking place at the pediatric hospital staffed by Christians, but the greatest miracle is undoubtedly the center itself. Conceived in the early 1970s when I was in Cambodia, it was completed in 1975 at a cost of about $750,000. Spending that much money for a capital investment in a country that seemed to have little or no future did not appear to be a very smart thing to do. I was frequently reminded of that by friends whose logic and reasoning were indisputable.

I could only answer, somewhat lamely, "But God has opened the door and we cannot fail to step through it." To me it was not an insignificant factor that a Buddhist country, which had thrown pastors and evangelists into jail just three years before, had now given seven acres of choice land just across the street from the National University to a Christian organization as the site for a children's hospital.

Our involvement in the country's agony had brought many opportunities for Christian witness and evangelism. To have backed away in the face of uncertainty would have destroyed our credibility and confirmed us as only fair-weather friends.

Nonetheless, I felt I needed some sure word from the Lord that our costly venture was not without His blessing. Clearly, the Holy Spirit directed me to Ecclesiastes 11. The chapter begins with a challenge to risk: "Cast thy bread upon the waters: for thou shalt find it after many days." I found assurance in verse four: "He that observeth the wind shall not sow; and he that regardeth the clouds shall not reap," or as *The Living Bible* paraphrases it: "If you wait for perfect conditions, you will never get anything done."

But the events of April, 1975, seemed to mock the promise. The hospital had been completed, equipment was in place, staff had arrived in Bangkok—and then the country gave up to the Khmer Rouge. When we had to evacuate, the hospital had never been used for even one day.

It was a bitter blow.

My last sight of the hospital was three days before

Phnom Penh fell. Using a chartered plane from Bangkok, we were flying daily into Pochentong airport—even then it was under constant rocket attack—with five tons of milk powder for our nutrition centers. On the return flights, we were bringing out abandoned babies that had been left in our care.

On our last takeoff from Pochentong, with 21 babies aboard, I asked the pilot to fly over the hospital which was near the airport. As I spotted the red tile roof glowing in the late afternoon sun, God gave me a supernatural peace that calmed my troubled spirit. He seemed to say, "Don't be anxious. Everything is under my control."

From that moment, I can honestly say that deep inside I knew that hospital would one day fulfill its original purpose. I remembered 1 Corinthians 15:58: "For you know that nothing you do for the Lord is ever wasted" (*TLB*).

The wait was four-and-a-half years. During that time, there was never any visible evidence to support my faith. Then in 1979, the Vietnamese army drove out Pol Pot, I was allowed to return to the new Kampuchea, and unexpectedly the government of Heng Samrin—although it was also Communist—offered to return the hospital.

It had, without doubt, been God's doing.

The hospital is still the newest building in Cambodia's capital city and, while it had been stripped inside, the building itself had suffered no structural damage. It was totally filthy, having been used by the genocidal Pol Pot as a torture chamber for dissenting intellectuals whom he had enticed with false promises to return from their exile in France.

After three steam cleanings, four months of construction work and nearly a million dollars, the hospital was opened in October, 1980. The new cornerstone carries the words: *Jesus said: "Let the children come to me,"* and the hospital was dedicated for the healing of children in His name. Many gentle miracles have since happened there.

The Communist government approved five senior staff positions for Christian personnel. They were supported by the 70 Khmer medical, administrative and service personnel.

When I was there, the mothers with their babies started arriving before seven o'clock in the morning. Before the day was over, the doctors would have treated well over 200 children. Since the people have nothing, no one is asked to pay either for the treatment or the medicines.

Ten very sick children had to be admitted as bed patients the first day I was there. Dr. Raley remarked, "If we don't get some discharges this afternoon, we'll be putting beds out in the hallway." Every bed has been full almost every night since the hospital was opened.

By midafternoon, one bed was empty, but it wasn't the kind of discharge the medic had in mind. I stepped into a ward where doctors and nurses were working frantically over the body of a child, using oxygen and heart massage in a vain attempt to restore life to a small girl who had stopped breathing. After 10 or 15 minutes, the oxygen was removed and a nurse pulled a sheet over the still form.

The parents sobbed inconsolably. Two other brothers clung to the weeping mother as she breast-fed a tiny infant. Other mothers in the ward, standing protectively over their own sick children, shed sympathizing tears. Sorrow filled us all.

The child who died was four years old and weighed only 15 pounds. I felt very empty and sad as the father gathered up the tiny bundle wrapped in a sheet and the sobbing family followed him down the hallway and out the door.

One of the Khmer nurses fainted dead away when the

child died, so the medical staff turned their attention to her. It is not the first time she has fainted, Dr. Raley told me. He can find nothing wrong with the woman and suspects that after seeing so much death during the times of Pol Pot, her mind and emotions now simply refuse to accept any more suffering. The little girl's death had triggered once again the pent-up hysteria with which she had lived for over four years.

The doctor tells me he has seen other severe psychological problems among the hospital staff. At first, several of the nurses were apathetic about the patients. All of their activity was mechanical, as if they didn't care whether the children lived or died. He is convinced that all their problems have their roots in the insane years of the nation's genocide when an estimated 2 million people were killed or cynically allowed to die.

One of the senior nurses lost her entire family, except a younger brother and her two daughters, six and nine. Her husband was a graduate medical student. Two brothers were professors and three more were prominent merchants.

When she came to work at the hospital, the doctor had to first treat her and her children for anemia and malnutrition. One day she came to him and complained about not being able to sleep.

"All the time I think about my family," she said. "You know doctor, for me it's finished, it's finished. There is no hope and nothing to live for."

Dr. Raley felt he was getting a clue that helped explain the nurse's apathy. He talked to her about her two children and how she had to live for them. His regular talks with her and some medication started her on the road to recovery. Gradually, he watched her and the other nurses go through a transformation from automatons into caring people. Later, his senior nurse insisted on working during a three-day national holiday. He tried to get her to take off just to rest, if not to celebrate.

She declined, saying, "No, my work is here. This is where I can help my people." She has accepted a Gospel of John and is reading it. The doctor believes a spiritual experience will also help her take another step toward complete psychological recovery.

Rarely does the hospital staff have the luxury of treating children with only one disease. Take measles, for example. This fairly routine children's disease in most of the world is a deadly killer here. As he examines a five-year-old girl who has measles—*Kampuchean* measles, he emphasizes—Dr. Raley explains why. "Malnutrition is the villain that turns measles into a killer," he told me. "Since almost all the children we see are first of all malnourished, they have a lot of complications. This girl came in at the point of death from profound pneumonia. Her lungs were full of fluid and infection. She had purulent conjunctivitis, profound anemia, pharyngitis and her liver was enlarged from an overwhelming load of parasites. In this case, it was hookworm.

"Frequently, a child also will have meningitis and/or malaria. Then if they have tuberculosis on top of that, as many do, they simply die. We just can't cope with those combinations compounded by malnutrition," Dr. Raley continued.

"Fortunately, it looks like we're ahead of this girl's problems. But if we didn't have this hospital and the mother had simply taken her to one of the local dispensaries, she would have been given maybe three tetracycline tablets and a couple of aspirin to treat the pneumonia. Eventually, the other untreated diseases would likely have killed her," he concluded.

So this hospital, the most modern one in the country, which might be just one of several options available to parents in any developed nation, stands here in Kampuchea as the last hope before death for thousands of children.

For some who arrive too late, and some do, it is the last stop on their way to an unmarked grave. At 5:45 in the evening, almost 11 hours after the staff started to treat the first patient of the day, two boys are brought in from Prey Veng, about 60 miles from Phnom Penh. Dr. André checks them over quickly and sends them to two different wards. A man, the father of 12-year-old Chhlonh, has brought them both. His son is grotesquely swollen and the father says he has been sick for five months.

I asked Dr. Raley what he thought might be wrong with the boy and he rattled off a string of 8 or 10 different medical terms. When I asked for a layman's translation, he said, "It could be thyroid failure, pancreatic failure, rupture of his lymph vessels, rupture of his bladder or some sort of leakage problem from his kidneys or renal failure. Whatever else is wrong, I know he has severe kwashiorkor (protein deficiency resulting from malnutrition).

"If this boy were at a hospital in the States, the workup alone would be massive. His initial orders would have $3,000 worth of laboratory tests, but since we're limited here, I have to go almost totally on my clinical impressions. I think he has a condition called nephrotic syndrome in which protein seeps out through a malfunctioning kidney. You would probably call it kidney failure.

"I don't give him more than a 50-50 chance."

I went to search out the other boy. Chhlonh's father told me the boy was an orphan, 11 years old, and his name was Pros. Dr. André told me Pros had severe kwashiorkor and bad burns on his legs. The rest of the diagnosis would have to be done the next day. That's all we knew about him.

Pros was lying on his ragged mat with a dirty pillow

under his head. The mat had been placed on a bed. His eyes were open, but unmoving and I couldn't see him breathing. There was no pulse and his hand was cold.

I called a nurse over. She also tested the vital signs, then looked at me and shook her head. Having gone through the hell of Pol Pot, I thought, Pros was finally at peace. But I was sorry he had to die before he could live. I took the filthy old blanket that had accompanied him and covered the body.

Even though no one was going to record the time of his death, instinctively I looked at my watch. It was a quarter past six in the evening. Outside it was getting dark.

I went to find one of the doctors. Dr. Raley was in the ward with the infants—"0 to 6 months" the sign said. With two nurses, he was working on a tiny baby only three months old. A light had been turned directly on the crib and by its glow he was trying to find a vein to continue the intravenous feeding on which the infant's life depends. The doctor has been at the hospital 12 hours and has been working over this child for almost an hour, but his hands are still steady.

He senses my presence and starts to talk while probing with the needle. "This baby has sepsis," he says, "which means that bacteria have blown out the blood vessels and capillaries. His blood pressure is so low that I can't find a vein, but I might not be able anyhow since he's so puffy.

"He was operated on for a blocked intestine by the East German team. It is a very sophisticated surgery and especially on a child this small. He went into cardiac arrest and had to be resuscitated. They brought him back here in shock and we had to resuscitate him again. We didn't expect him to live more than three or four hours, but it's been nine days.

"It looks like they'll need to do remedial surgery

tomorrow, so I've got to keep this kid hydrated tonight. I thought I had a vein in the scalp a few minutes ago, but it wouldn't take the drip. We've used every one of his veins and I really don't want to cut down on his wrist (a procedure where tissue is cut to expose a vein) because that may be the only lifeline the doctors have during the operation.

"So I've got to resort to an emergency measure. I learned it in the Amazon with dehydrated babies because the hospitals were too dirty and there were too many flies to do cutdowns. It's a primitive procedure that would never be done in a hospital in the United States because the surgeon would simply do an incision and put a central line right into the heart.

"But since I'm not a surgeon, I'll try something else. We'll pray that it works."

I watch fascinated, praying all the while.

Dr. Raley feels along the baby's leg with a doctor's educated touch. Finding the right point, he then takes a needle and pushes it into the leg below the kneecap. He keeps pressing and turning the needle until it stands rigid. He attaches a syringe and draws a few drops of blood.

The needle has penetrated the bone into the marrow!

"The bone marrow is the most vascular part of the body and will absorb very easily," he tells me. "Given this baby's problems, a possible infection from this procedure is a very small risk."

The IV tube is attached and the drip starts. The leg is splinted and we leave little Bora for the night. The next morning, his blood vessels have expanded and the German team comes early to repair the surgery.

A photographer traveling with me, Jon Kubly, gets a chance to give a pint of his type 0 blood before he shoots the operation. He took pictures of his own blood dripping into the tiny infant.

As we prepare to leave the house of healing and hope a couple of hours after the surgery, baby Bora is holding his own. Medical skill, compassion and prayer have all combined to give him a fighting chance. Considering his capacity for survival, the doctors think his chance is a better than even one.

On my way out, I went to say good-bye to our other survivor, Chap. He is still pulling his toy train up and down the hallway. As I turn to leave, I wave

Chap smiles.

Just one more gentle miracle.

12

A Disturbing Silence

Ethiopia

They sat so quietly that it bothered me.

It was the first real food most of them had seen for months. Nothing more formidable than a bramble fence separated them from the sacks of grain that had arrived the previous day. Yet they watched without moving while relief workers carefully rationed out the grain to those inside the enclosure—the lucky ones who had arrived earlier and had managed to get their names on the distribution list.

Many more were outside the makeshift fence—at least 2,000. "Why don't they rush the handful of guards and take the food?" I thought to myself. "What have they got to lose?"

Maybe they were resigned to approaching death. Or too weak and tired to protest. Or simply beyond caring.

I knew only that I could emotionally handle a riot better than their disturbing silence. Yet I've learned from working with the starving on every continent: first, violence is virtually unknown among them and, second, they go to their graves mostly uncomplaining.

The Srumah people of Ethiopia were validating what I had seen everywhere else, and I was devastated by it.

I was back in the country early in 1981, just four months after an initial survey of the drought-stricken areas. My eyes had confirmed reports of millions of people seriously affected by hunger. On the earlier trip we had flown an antiquated DC-3 right down into the desert area of Gamo-Gofa province where Kenya, Sudan and Ethiopia share a common border.

There I had talked to the Bume tribespeople and learned of the tragedy of the past three years during which the rains had failed. They told of the death of all their cattle which meant the loss of their sole livelihood.

Now we were in Kaffa province in Srumah (where coffee is a principal crop and from where the beverage gets its name), another of the nine areas affected by what *Newsweek* magazine called "the worst drought in fifteen years." The people here had suffered badly.

The trip to Srumah is a journey down and back, both geographically and symbolically. First, you go down. The plateau which is the seat of Ethiopia's capital, Addis Ababa, and the provincial center, Jimma, drops suddenly from over 7500 feet to less than 2500 feet, down to Africa's Rift Valley. A ruggedly beautiful escarpment marks the line. The color goes from green to brown.

Once you are off the escarpment, the journey is also back. Back in time. The nomadic Srumah people still live in the early Stone Age. Even the use of the wheel is unknown to them. For centuries their life has been ordered by the seasons as they have moved their cattle back and forth across the baking hot lowlands in search of grass and water.

It is hard for an urban sophisticate in the Western world to understand what cattle mean to the nomads. Here where we breed and feed beef only for the market, we cannot comprehend the emotional and personal feelings a nomadic herder has for his cattle. He slaughters one only for the most festive and ceremonious occasion.

He milks them, bleeds them (mixing the blood with maize meal), tends them, makes up songs about them, uses them to buy wives and passes the herd down to his sons. A wealthy man may have thousands of head of cattle. They are not only the source of his life; they *are* his life. During this current drought, one man lost all his cattle but two. He had to drive that remaining pair a long way to find water, but before the animals could drink, they fell dead, at the very edge of the river. The cattle herder was so overcome with grief that he tried to commit suicide on the spot.

When drought occurs, the order of death among the nomadic herders is this: First the cattle. Next the young children. Followed by the aged ones. Then the lactating mothers. Finally the rest of the adults. The unrelenting sequence occurs with awful regularity among the nomads of East Africa.

The desperate plight of the Srumah people was signaled to me as soon as the plane taxied to the end of the dirt runway. Usually one can expect large numbers of people to provide an enthusiastic welcome when the visitors step off the airplane. It didn't happen at Srumah. Almost no one followed the plane down the strip, and the greetings exchanged when the engines shut down were somber and subdued.

It didn't take me long to learn why. There is little enthusiasm for anything in a place where the people are dying from hunger at the rate of nearly one an hour.

As I walked back down toward the distribution point, I saw something that threatened to do me in. A younger woman was helping her old mother walk to the place where food would be available. The old woman walked a few steps and then collapsed on the ground, literally a pile of skin and bones. The frail body, the tattered rags that covered it, the hopeless resignation mirrored in her face, the fact that motherhood and age were reduced to such final indignity—it was almost more than I could bear.

Since she was too weak to lift herself, some of us took her to the thatch building nearby and sat her down on the ground against a wall, next to a woman equally bad off. It looked like neither of them could have weighed more than 60 or 65 pounds.

I talked to her daughter. She and her sister and her aged widowed mother came here two days before from the bush. They had not yet been able to get registered for food allocation—1 and when there is an allocation. Because the daughters are not married there were few cattle for them even in the better years. In normal times, however, when there was rain the women scratched out a subsistence garden. Since even poverty has its ranks, these women would have been the poorest among the poor.

But now hunger has become the common denominator of all Srumah society. In this camp of 11,000 people, I saw scores of men and women in the final stages of starvation. Only when the Cambodians were fleeing to Thailand after four years of Pol Pot's tyranny had I seen so many adults as bad off as the old people of Srumah.

Then I remembered the Grim Reaper's priority list. First the cattle. Next the children. Then the old ones. It seemed I was already looking at stage three.

But as I looked around, I saw that death was not yet through with the infants. Right behind me, a young mother was cradling in her arms one of the most emaciated babies I had ever seen. Even if the mother's breasts had not been empty, the baby was too weak to nurse. It appeared, in fact, to be already in a coma. The woman told me she was a widow and the mother of four children. One of her children was already dead. I was certain that not even her anxious love could keep death away long from the 10-month-old baby enfolded tenderly in her arms and over which she protectively arched her body.

As we turned away, an Ethiopian colleague wept openly. Sure enough, the camp assistant came just before we left to tell us about the baby's death. That means, I thought, she has only half of her children remaining.

Death visits the Srumah camp almost hourly. No one knows how frequently the dark angel comes to the families living in the bush a day's walk away. Likely, with at least equal regularity, meaning that the 27,000 Srumah people—less than half of whom are in the camp—are dying at the rate of between 30 and 50 a day.

For centuries the Srumah have survived without outside help. They are a proud race of survivors. But since the rains started to fail in 1971, the people have been pushed to the edge of extinction. The most recent drought may be the *coup de grace* for this threatened people.

One tribal leader told me: "We have become beggars because of nature. We do not want to be like that but have no choice. We must ask for help."

Another tribal leader hobbled over to where we were talking. His white hair and white wisp of a beard distinguished him from the others. His legs were swollen and his ankles were puffy and scaly—obvious signs of malnutrition. He could stand only with the aid of his walking stick, but he proudly refused the supporting arm of a younger man who offered it to him. I had the feeling that he wanted to talk to me on his own two feet.

Managing the business of interpretation in a situation like this was not easy. The people did not even speak Amharic, the language of the country's majority, and there was no one who could translate directly from Srumah to

English. So we had to go from Srumah to Amharic to English, and then back again over the same linguistic route.

I knew so much was being lost in this process, especially the feeling behind the words I so desperately wished to experience. But even with this inadequate procedure, his words were still starkly eloquent: "We appeal to the world through you. We have nothing to put on. We're cold.

"Our old people and our children are dying out. I see people dying every day. We are surrounded by graves. We really need help. We need food, but we also need seed to plant. Unless we get food immediately, we will all die."

A young man spoke up: "This is our old father. Our mother couldn't come here today because she is too weak. There are so many more out there who can't walk to this place. Please help us."

Even as the young man spoke, I could not take my eyes off his father. The old man's eyes—clear, convicting, compelling—riveted me to the spot and would not release me until I made a response. What I said sounded so inadequate for the desperate moment: "Your words touch my heart. I have seen much suffering today. I wish we could save the life of every old person and every child, but I cannot make false promises. You know so many are already beyond help.

"However, working together with your government and the Relief Commission, I promise you that we will not allow the Srumah people to die as a race."

He said simply, "Please do your best as soon as possible."

Then his eyes released me.

As we moved away, others approached me. I did not understand their words, but the gestures of patting the stomach and putting fingers to the mouth were unmistakable. For the moment, I had nothing to give and was unable to respond beyond a warm clasp of the hand or an encouraging pat on the shoulder. To starving people, the gestures must have been as empty as I felt inside.

I was saved emotionally from this moment as the camp director came to tell us that a few hundred yards away they would bury an old man who had died that morning. Several burials had already taken place that day. It seemed to be a never-ending ritual.

As we made our way toward the burial site, we passed through an area where stones had been formed into small mounds to hold cooking pots. Most of the people who used to stay out here in the open, I was told, had now gone back into the bush or over into Sudan. There they find grass, leaves and acorns to eat. Here there has been no food to distribute. Yesterday's relief flight was the first in two months.

We arrived at the place of burial before the grave was finished. It was simply an oval hole about three feet deep. The man digging it looked fairly robust. An official informed me that those who dig graves and handle dead bodies are given special rations, since custom forbids them to live with their families for a period of time. Because of the many deaths here, those engaged in this work live alone all the time.

Three months ago, the official said, the young man digging this grave came here very emaciated. He agreed to take on the burial task in order to get the extra food. Now his well-fed appearance is in such contrast with the others that he looks as if he came from some other place.

Soon the body arrived, tied up in cowhide and lashed to a pole carried by two men. The family—stepmother, daughter, son-in-law and two grandchildren—came with the corpse. Custom dictated that the widow remain at the shelter in mourning.

There were no last words, no eulogy, no prayer. The

only ritual performed, as far as I could tell, was twofold. The grandchildren each had a small rattle tied to a wrist, and their mother encouraged them to shake these constantly over the body. Just before the body was placed in the grave—on its side and drawn up in the fetal position— the daughter poured a small amount of milk from a gourd into both ears. If this is not done, tradition has it, other members of the family will die.

No friends were present. I never learned if this was because it was the custom or if death had become so commonplace that going to burials had become impractical. I suspect it was the latter.

As we returned to camp, the people who had been waiting and hoping for some grain were returning to their little open air campsites with empty gourds. If they ate anything today, it would be the usual grass and acorns, although even that was becoming in short supply around the camp.

There had been no riot, no ugly protest. Not even any shouting. The quiet dignity with which the Srumah people were suffering under the onslaught of nature and the indifference of the rest of the human family was like a stab wound in my own conscience.

I gathered a few of the tribal leaders together and told them that we planned to purchase an airplane in order to get food to them as quickly as possible. To help them connect the plane with my visit—and so they wouldn't think I was simply a tourist who came to view their suffering with no intention of helping—I told them the plane would bear a symbol of a cross over a globe.

"When you see that painting on the airplane," I said, "you will know I have kept my promise."

Once again they thanked me.

As we climbed into the ancient DC-3 and headed up to the plateau, leaving all the sadness below, my Ethiopian colleague told me what had caused him to cry when we saw that starving infant. The previous night, he said, he had to make a decision about our box lunches for the next day. He had to choose whether he would get them from the hotel where we were staying or from an airlines catering service. The big question he faced was, "Which would be the most pleasing?"

As he looked at the baby near death from starvation, he suddenly remembered making that choice. Knowing that baby had no choice, even between life and death, he felt shame and grief and couldn't hold back the tears.

I nodded my head in understanding.

It is not a strange feeling to those who run rescue shops so close to hell.

13
The Shared Canteen

Whatever you believe and however deeply you believe it amounts to nothing more than pious idealism if it doesn't cause something to happen in your life. Religious faith has got to lead to something, demand something, produce something. Otherwise, why believe?

The Christian religion, which has at its central core the incarnational language of "the Word becoming flesh" is, in this twentieth century, in danger of reversing the incarnational process. We are turning flesh into words.

You're not sure about that? Try a simple experiment. Check out the next 10 church conventions you hear about. What did the delegates do? Most likely, they took "actions." And what were those actions? Resolutions, declarations, protests, affirmations, conclusions—all verbal and none requiring anything more than a raised hand or a spoken vote.

Actions? "Sittings" would be a more accurate word to describe them. One delegate reported back to his church, "We deplored, we decried and we departed."

In religion we have done very well with our *whereases*,

our *thusly's,* and our *namely's,* but we have neglected our *therefores*—those adverbial connectors between faith and life, between belief and action.

My convictions and beliefs, though they are a necessary basis for what I do, don't really matter much, even to me, if they do not result in something happening.

In his treatise on practical religion, the Apostle James argues: "My brothers, what use is it for a man to say he has faith when he does nothing to show it? Can that faith save him? Suppose a brother or sister is in rags with not enough food for the day, and one of you says, 'Good luck to you, keep yourselves warm, and have plenty to eat,' but does nothing to supply their bodily needs, what is the good of that? So with faith; if it does not lead to action, it is in itself a lifeless thing" (Jas. 2:14-17, *NEB*). James is not denigrating belief. He is simply affirming what I affirm: Believing must be translated into living.

For James and me, beliefs are basic. They are the givens that make everything else possible. Archimedes is supposed to have said, "Give me a place to stand and a lever long enough and I will move the earth." A place to stand is very important if you expect to do much moving. Where I stand is on my confession as a follower of the Way, an evangelical Christian, born again by the Spirit of God and expecting the triumphant return of Jesus Christ to establish His Kingdom with power and justice.

The place where I stand is compassed by my belief that this world is, by right of ownership, God's world. Because I believe in God, it follows naturally that I must believe in humanity, that unique part of God's creation made in His image. Believing that God is for man, not against him, I must care about my fellow human beings in their deprived and oppressed physical condition as well as in their alienated and lost spiritual state. That makes it impossible for me to limit my concern to their spiritual needs while ignoring their other problems.

My beliefs have taken me often, and for extended periods, among the dispossessed, the hungry, the disfranchised of our world. For His own sovereign reason, God has not called me to share their lot, but He has called me to plead their cause, to champion their hopes, to identify with their aspirations.

The hell-on-earth where so many of my fellow humans live is populated by the hungry, the illiterate, the homeless, the oppressed, the hopeless. That describes about half the people on this planet. Their world embraces 800 million severely malnourished people, 17 million children who will die this year because no one cares enough to give $100 per child to save them, and 12 million refugees who have no homeland, no future and marginal hope.

It is a world where statistics have faces and where numbers have names. It is a world where little children ask the twisted question, "Is there life *before* death?"

It is a world from which I, as a Christian, may not live detached. At various times in my pilgrimage of faith I have read statements and affirmations that have helped me translate my beliefs into compassionate action. Three of them have provided special motivation.

The first is an ancient Chinese proverb that, I believe, has compelling contemporary application. It says, "Of all precious things on earth, the most precious is people."

No other resource on this planet, of whatever short supply, is of such value as human life. I am aware of the endangered status of the gray whale, the Bengal tiger, the black rhinoceros and the bald eagle, and I am not indifferent to the loss in our natural environment which their disappearance would cause. But my passion must at least equal that of the environmentalists when I ask: "Who will make the speeches and organize the movements on behalf of my brothers and sisters threatened by famine, disease, poverty and injustice?" Is human life so cheap, especially if it is not white-skinned, that it is no longer a cause worth championing? Does not our common humanity—to say nothing of our Christian commitment—call from us something that protects the weak and helpless, the downtrodden and powerless?

For myself, I hold dual citizenship—on earth and in heaven. My earthly citizenship as a member of the human family was not canceled when, through faith in Jesus Christ, I took on a heavenly citizenship. Rather, the second enhanced the first. Now it seems the nearer I come to the person of Jesus Christ, the closer I feel to suffering humanity. Or is it the other way around? I'm not sure. I haven't got that part of it sorted out yet. I know only that one day I saw people as whole persons, not just disembodied souls, and my view of man—and of God—was perceptibly heightened.

Every person has intrinsic worth because he or she is made in the image of God. The Marxist view of man is that he has value only so long as he produces for the State. That is why in some Communist countries the only social service permitted to the Church is to care for the mentally retarded or the elderly. Those lives have less value in the eyes of the State than, say, children in an orphanage. The old or mentally deficient have no potential for producing. But with what tender care have I seen the loving hands of Christ's people minister to those who are without worth or value in a materialistic society!

When I see preachers and assorted religious leaders engaging in political power plays, I can't help asking myself if Jesus would be stalking the corridors of an empire, currying favor with the big and powerful, or would He still be walking dusty paths with the poor? The question is rhetorical, since the answer is self-evident.

Recently, I came across a book, *Portrait of Jesus* (New

York: Mayflower Books, 1979), by an Englishman named Alan T. Dale. I don't know if Mr. Dale shares my evangelical convictions, but I resonate to some of the conclusions he formed after drawing in words his personal portrait of Jesus.

Citing those who are overlooked, neglected and scorned in today's society—the man or woman who is left out of the picture, the one nobody bothers with, that person who doesn't seem "to belong," the individual who is always left "out of it," Dale states what Jesus made clear to him: that "there can be no genuine human society if anybody is left out." Therefore, to leave anybody out is to corrupt human society and destroy it.

Dale's study of the life of Christ brought home to him the realization that Jesus did not talk just about being "kind" and "generous," but rather about how a world can ever be a world in any true sense of the word unless the whole human family is included at the dinner table.

For me, those thoughts have profound application.

A few years ago, when the refugees were streaming into India out of Bangladesh to escape the civil war, I drove from Calcutta to the border over roads choked by the fleeing families. An estimated 200,000 people were on the roads that hot, sticky day. As we moved slowly through the masses of people, I saw the crumpled body of an old woman lying in a ditch. Assuming she was dead, we drove on. When we returned an hour later, I saw that she was moving about and moaning. The thin cotton *sari* she had been wearing earlier had been stripped from her body even before she had stopped breathing.

I asked the driver to stop, and I went down into the ditch. The woman was alive but very sick and incoherent. In order to cover her nakedness, I bought a piece of cloth from another refugee and wrapped it around her.

One of my companions joined me and we carried her

across the road to a temporary camp where I tried to get the director to take her in. He refused, saying he had no hospital or medical facilities for one so obviously near death. I offered to leave money and pay someone just to bring her water and food twice a day until she died, but I could find no takers.

In desperation, I got the camp commander to give me a little thatched lean-to that was empty. I bought a bamboo mat, and we laid her on it in the shade of the tiny shelter. She ate some bread and drank a few sips of water. After putting the rest of the water and bread beside her, we had to leave.

There was nothing more I could do.

But I was haunted by that scene. We had done so little. Was it all an empty symbolism, meaningless in the face of such remaining awesome needs? Should those few moments and few rupees have been spent on someone with a better chance of survival?

I know the answer. No life is valueless, even one so near death. If Mother Teresa is right—and she is—when she says, "When we minister to the poor, we minister to Christ," then we had cared for Jesus that day, as simple as our act of love had been.

I believe the Master would affirm what the Chinese say, "Of all precious things on earth, the most precious is people."

The second statement that drives me back into action when I want to quit is something I read many years ago from Aristotle. I stumbled onto it during a freshman literature course and was so profoundly moved by it that I wrote it on the flyleaf of the first Bible I ever owned. What Aristotle said is both simple and deep: "Where there are things to be done, the end is not to survey and recognize those various things, but rather to do them."

Somehow, I never felt that God was offended to have a

Greek philosopher quoted on one of the blank pages of my Bible. Why should He be since He is the source of all truth, no matter where it comes from?

I think God would affirm Aristotle's statement, too, since He has proven Himself throughout history to be the God who acts. Aristotle is saying that it is not enough to research, analyze, synthesize and hypothesize when human life and dignity are at stake. That is not to say that those things shouldn't be done at all, but there comes a crucial moment when all those things must be finished, the nettle grasped, the action begun.

Have you ever taken a side or made a decision when you wished you had more information or more time? Of course you have. The evidence is never all in. The time comes, in any case, when a judgment has to be made. After logic has done its best, there is still a gap that only the heart can bridge. History moves over that last gap, not upon reason, but upon the action, at risk, of a person who determines that, come what may, he must do right.

History's grandest moments also have been history's moments of greatest risk. The *great* leader does not wait until advocacy is safe. Anwar Sadat may have been the best contemporary example of such courageous leadership when he went to Jerusalem in an attempt to break the stalemate and hostility between Egypt and Israel.

A person does not become a leader by searching out a cause. He becomes a leader by daring to do what must be done.

As a young member of the British Parliament, William Wilberforce was converted to Christ while on a trip to France in 1787. He returned to London, hoping to take holy orders, but was dissuaded by the hymn writer and former slave captain, John Newton, who urged him to serve his Lord in the House of Commons.

Wilberforce agreed and determined to use his office to

attack not only the slave trade but the very institution of slavery itself. He was a leader in that fight for the rest of his life. It took 20 years of struggle, but when his vision was finally caught by younger members of Parliament, the bill to abolish slave traffic was carried in 1807 by a vote of 283 to 6. It took another 26 years before 700,000 slaves were permanently freed throughout the empire, and it didn't happen until a month after Wilberforce died. But his name shines lustrous in England's history.

One of the great moral challenges facing the world today is Third-World poverty and injustice. It is a just and right cause that languishes for lack of strong voices and committed leadership. It is time for Christians to hear the words of Aristotle: "Where there are things to be done, the end is not to survey and recognize those various things, but rather to do them."

The last principle that constantly challenges me comes from Jesus. But first, let me tell you about an experience.

In a park in Atlanta, Georgia, there is a large circular building in which is portrayed the battle that once raged around that city during the Civil War. The exhibit in the Cyclorama is realistic—partly shown on a huge circular canvas and partly by means of three-dimensional figures that occupy the foreground, some of the figures projecting from the painting itself. So cleverly is the portrayal done that it is difficult to tell where the three-dimensional figures end and the painting begins. It is almost like participatory theater.

I joined about 50 other visitors as we took our seats on an elevated central core. As it started to revolve, a narrator told us the story of the Battle of Atlanta. Each scene would light up in synchronization with the account.

Here the Confederates have broken through a cut in the rail line to attack a beleaguered squad of Union soldiers. There a detail of Southern prisoners is being marched away. From the top of a hill, General William Sherman watches, astride his horse.

Close to the railroad, a stone wall forms a barricade behind which the Confederate troops deploy, so close to the enemy that it becomes a hand-to-hand struggle. Two figures in this group are illuminated, a soldier in blue who is bent over a soldier in gray.

"These are the Martin brothers from Tennessee," our hushed group heard the narrator say. "One enlisted to fight for the Union and the other for the Confederacy. They never communicated after that. In the midst of the battle, this Union soldier stops to lift his canteen to the lips of a dying Southern boy who is pleading for water. As he puts his arm under the head of the fallen soldier to raise it for a drink, he discovers that the dying youth is . . . his brother."

There is silence. The illusion has been so real and the concentration so intense that we seem to have been standing on a vantage point looking down into the carnage where men are struggling desperately, where blood is pooling from their shattered bodies, and shrill cries of shell-torn horses pierce the air.

Then the spell is broken. Fifty silent people walk out into daylight.

Many times as I move through our broken and fractured world, I think of that scene. So many have been wounded by life, felled by poverty, plagued by hunger, victimized by injustice, brutalized by sin. And then I see those of us who stand upright with full canteens. Do we know who is at our feet, crying out with thirst? Do we wait to make sure he is a brother before we help? Or might it be that in the giving of a drink of water or the helping hand or the healing word or the shared loaf or the redemptive act we will discover our brother?

Here is what Jesus said about it. It is clear and direct,

needing no commentary: "Anything you did for one of my brothers here, however humble, you did for me" (Matt. 25:40, *NEB*).

Perhaps kinship is recognized through an act of serving love. I know without doubt that every single act of kindness is blessed by Christ to both receiver and giver. Jesus makes a lavish promise: "Whoever gives a cup of cold water in my name shall not lose his reward" (see Matt. 10:42). When we do what lies at hand, when we do what we can do, we can count on Christ to bless and reward the effort because we are living by His giving principle.

Some time ago, Mother Teresa told me a story that underscores this truth beautifully. She said she had returned from receiving the Nobel Peace Prize which carried, I think, a cash award of over $100,000. She gave it all to her religious order in Calcutta, the Missionaries of Charity. Back on the streets of that distressed Indian city, she came upon a beggar who recognized her and pressed a 10-paisa coin in her hand. In United States money, it was one cent.

"Now that you have all that money," he told her, "you don't need my gift. But I need to give it."

There is a secret in there somewhere. I need to give, not so much because others need to receive, but because the experience of giving will change me.

There are so many brothers and sisters hungering and thirsting, wandering and wasting, waiting to be found. I am not optimistic that the world will ever be without poverty, hunger and injustice. However, I do believe if we can get enough people to replicate the caring act of the shared canteen or any modern equivalent of the cup of cold water in Jesus' name, you and I can make a difference in our world.

I know that, for me, I can't stop trying.

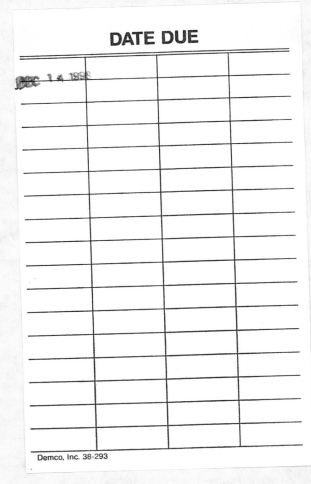

DATE DUE

DEC 1 4 1998			